Manual
of
Gerontologic
Nursing

Manual of Gerontologic Nursing

CHARLOTTE ELIOPOULOS,
R.N.C., M.P.H., C.D.O.N.A./L.T.C.

Consultant in Private Practice
Baltimore, Maryland

with 57 illustrations

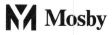 Mosby

St. Louis Baltimore Berlin Boston Carlsbad Chicago London Madrid
Naples New York Philadelphia Sydney Tokyo Toronto

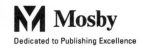

Mosby

Dedicated to Publishing Excellence

Editor: Michael S. Ledbetter
Developmental Editor: Teri Merchant
Project Manager: John Rogers
Senior Production Editor: Helen Hudlin
Designer: Renée Duenow
Manufacturing Supervisor: Theresa Fuchs
Copyright © 1995 by Mosby-Year Book, Inc.

Printed in the United States of America
Composition by University Graphics, Inc.
Printing/binding by R.R. Donnelly

Mosby–Year Book, Inc.
11830 Westline Industrial Drive
St. Louis, Missouri 63146

Library of Congress Cataloging-in-Publication Data

Eliopoulos, Charlotte.
    Manual of gerontologic nursing / Charlotte Eliopoulos.
       p.   cm.
    Includes bibliographical references and index.
    ISBN 0-8016-7994-X
    1. Geriatric nursing—Handbooks, manuals, etc.   I. Title.
    [DNLM: 1. Geriatric Nursing—handbooks.   2. Nursing Diagnosis—handbooks. WT 39 E42m   1994]
    RC954.E463   1994
    610.73'65--dc 20
    DNLM/DLC
    for Library of Congress   94-28513
                                        CIP

96 97 98 99 / 9 8 7 6 5 4 3 2

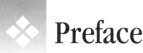

Preface

Nursing has a long history of caring for the elderly. Before it became popular or profitable for other professionals to become involved with the geriatric population, nurses assumed major responsibility for staffing institutions, taking services into the homes of older adults, and using their own homes to provide room, board, and personal care to the elderly as a forerunner to today's nursing home.

The unique aspects of nursing for the aged were not acknowledged in any significant degree until the 1960s. In 1961 the American Nurses' Association (ANA) recommended the development of a special interest group for geriatric nurses that led to the first national meeting of the Conference Group on Geriatric Nursing. In 1966 the ANA launched the Division of Geriatric Nursing, giving legitimacy to the specialty. Within the decade that followed, marked strides were made: Standards for Geriatric Nursing Practice emerged, certification in the specialty became available, literature in the field increased more than tenfold, and the division changed its name from *Geriatric* to *Gerontological Nursing* to reflect the broader scope of nursing's involvement with aging persons. The growth in the quality and quantity of gerontologic practitioners and the professionalization of the specialty have been steady since that time. Today the specialty of nursing the aged is receiving the credibility and respect it has long deserved.

The development of nursing diagnoses has followed a path similar to that of the specialty of gerontologic nursing. Nursing historically contributed to patient care but failed to describe that contribution in a manner that helped to differentiate it from medical practice. Through the 1960s and 1970s nurse theorists attempted to design nursing models, such as Roy's Adaptation Model, Orem's Self-Care Theory, and Roger's Life Processes. These nursing theories received lukewarm reception by many nurses who viewed them as too academic or irrelevant to their practice. Then came nursing diagnosis! When the National Group for the Classification of Nursing Diagnosis held its first meeting in 1973 there were skeptics ready to judge this effort as another academic exercise, but the momentum grew as did the number of nurses who understood the relevancy of nursing diagnosis to their practice. Nursing diagnosis made logical sense and meshed nicely into the nursing process that most nurses understood.

It is interesting that the advancement of gerontologic nursing and nursing diagnosis occurred within similar time frames although down separate paths, because when the major problems of the geriatric client are considered it is easy to see that they fall within the realm of nursing to diagnose and treat. Ask nurses who work with the elderly what problems consume their time and effort and the response will not be diabetes, congestive heart failure, cancer, or other medical diagnoses but the nursing diagnoses generated from them, such as the potential for injury, noncompliance, knowledge deficit, impaired physical mobility, and self-care deficits. Thus the marriage of gerontologic nursing and nursing diagnosis seems appropriate and natural.

The purpose of this book is to present major gerontologic nursing care problems within a nursing diagnosis framework. Practical information is presented in an easily retrievable format to offer guidance to nurses who wish to implement this framework into their practice. For the new user of nursing diagnosis, time and practice in using this approach may be required to gain comfort and skill in its use. However, once nurses incorporate nursing diagnosis into their practice, they will discover that it contributes to more organized care delivery, helps demonstrate nursing's unique practice realm, and provides a foundation for research and knowledge development.

This text is organized into three major parts. The first part reviews general facts about the older population and about gerontologic nursing, covering topics such as age-related changes, theories of aging, and assessment and care planning. The second part is the largest one and is dedicated to a review of the major functional health patterns. Within each chapter dedicated to a functional health pattern, the major nursing diagnoses related to the pattern are presented with discussions of the characteristics of the diagnosis, causative/contributing factors, clinical manifestations, assessment considerations, goal menu, nursing interventions, and evaluation criteria. Selected health problems related to nursing diagnoses are also included. The final part presents special care issues such as safe drug use, legal-ethical issues, and resources, and offers practical guidelines for gerontologic nurses. The intent is to provide information in a format that is easy to use and relevant to nurses who desire essential, basic information on a topic.

The specialty of gerontologic nursing has experienced tremendous growth in a relatively short time. The challenge now is to assist those who provide nursing services to older adults to use the wealth of knowledge that has been gained. Hopefully, this book will assist in bridging the gap between existing knowledge and the practitioner who needs that knowledge to provide high-quality gerontologic nursing care.

CHARLOTTE ELIOPOULOS

Contents

Part Three
Special Issues in Gerontologic Nursing Care

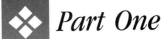

Part One

General
Considerations

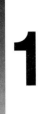

Nursing and the Aging

GERIATRICS, GERONTOLOGY, AND NURSING

Historically, the elderly and the aging process have always been of interest. As early as the sixth century BC, Taoism promoted old age as the epitome of life and a reflection of a tremendous accomplishment. During the fifth century BC, Confucius proposed that the greater one's age, the greater the honor and respect to which that person was entitled. In the centuries that followed, diverse reactions to old age and aging emerged. The early Egyptians invested considerable effort in seeking eternal youth. Plato advocated elders as society's leaders and recommended techniques for healthy aging, whereas Aristotle wished to exclude the elderly from important societal matters. Throughout the Dark Ages and Middle Ages the elderly held a low status and led difficult existences. Primarily in the twentieth century, increased numbers of old people and greater sensitivity to the needs of all human beings have caused the elderly to gain a new, positive recognition and enjoy a better life.

GERIATRICS VS. GERONTOLOGY

The terms *geriatrics* and *gerontology* often are used interchangeably although there is a difference in meaning. Geriatrics is the branch of medicine concerned with the illnesses of old age and their care. Gerontology is the scientific study of the factors affecting the normal aging process and the effects of aging on persons of all ages. In a true sense these terms are not synonymous.

Much of the past interest in gerontology revolved around interest in achieving immortality and eternal youth, witnessed by various potions and fountains of youth that were promoted at different times in history. Only in the last century has increasingly sophisticated research interest developed in learning about normal aging so that individuals could understand the way to age in a healthy manner. Findings such as the correlation of parents' longevity to their offspring's longevity and the importance of proper nutrition, exercise, rest, and stress management to healthy aging have been some of the outcomes of gerontologic research.

Nascher wrote the first gerontologic medicine textbook in 1914 but only in recent years has gerontology grown tremendously. In the past, many pathologic conditions (e.g., dementia, incontinence, immobility, and sexual dysfunction) were accepted as expected outcomes of growing old. Unique norms in vital signs and laboratory values were unknown, and the elderly were given unnecessary treatments to achieve norms for younger persons. It is fortunate that research findings have given insight into normal and pathologic conditions in late life, and appropriate, age-specific care measures have been and are still being developed.

One of the exciting aspects of gerontologic and geriatric care is that they are young, rapidly developing specialties. Professionals in this area are afforded an opportunity seldom available in other fields: the chance to influence the development of a specialty.

NURSING AND THE CARE OF THE ELDERLY

Long before it became a popular specialty, the care of the elderly was a responsibility and interest of nursing. Nurses were among the early care givers of the elderly in almshouses, asylums, chronic disease and other types of hospitals, nursing homes, and the community. In fact, the term *nursing home* stemmed from room-and-board houses operated by nurses or women who called themselves nurses. Geriatric nursing, because of the low status and salaries offered, was not a practice area that drew a great number of highly prepared or competent nurses. Often, nurses drawn to geriatric care were those who could not function well in other settings; thus the stigma associated with this specialty was perpetuated.

Nursing's long-standing concern with the unique needs of

the elderly is demonstrated by an article in a 1904 issue of the *American Journal of Nursing* in which the principles of caring for the aged were described (Bishop, 1904). However, it was not until the early 1960s that a specialty group for geriatric nurses was promoted by the American Nurses' Association (ANA). The years that followed brought significant growth for the specialty, as shown in Box 1-1.

Clinical research, teaching, and administrative leadership in this specialty have developed significantly as growing numbers of well-prepared, dynamic nurses are learning the challenges of working with the elderly.

However, just as the terms *gerontology* and *geriatrics* differ in meaning, geriatric nursing and gerontologic nursing also differ. Geriatric nursing focuses on the care of the sick aged, whereas gerontologic nursing includes health maintenance, illness prevention, illness management, and quality of life promotion to aid persons of all ages grow old in a state of optimum health and well-being. The scope of gerontologic nursing is broader than that of geriatric nursing.

BOX 1-1   Highlights in the Development of Gerontologic Nursing

1961 ANA recommended specialty group for geriatric nurses

1962 First national ANA Conference on Geriatric Nursing Practice

1966 Geriatric Nursing Division formed within ANA; Duke University launched first gerontologic nursing clinical specialist program

1970 ANA published standards for geriatric nursing practice

1975 ANA offered first certification for geriatric nursing practice; *Journal of Gerontological Nursing* published

1976 ANA Geriatric Nursing Division changed to Gerontological Nursing Division; ANA published *Standards for Gerontological Nursing Practice*

1981 ANA Division of Gerontological Nursing published statement, *Scope of Gerontological Nursing Practice*

1982 Robert Wood Johnson Teaching Nursing Home Program developed

1983 First chair in gerontologic nursing offered at Case Western Reserve University

1984 ANA Division on Gerontological Nursing Practice became Council on Gerontological Nursing

1986 National Association for Directors of Nursing Administration in Long-Term Care (NADONNA/LTC) formed

WHO ARE GERONTOLOGIC NURSES?

Only a small fraction of registered nurses are employed in geriatric facilities but that is not to imply that only a small number are working with the elderly. Nurses provide significant services to older adults in a variety of settings, including the following:

- *Acute hospitals.* Most hospitals find that a majority of their medical-surgical beds are filled by persons over 65 years of age. Hospital outpatient departments have replaced the community general practitioner as the source of medical care for increasing numbers of elderly.
- *Home health agencies.* The largest portion of home health agencies' clients are older adults. Reimbursement policies that discourage inpatient care have resulted in greater numbers of seriously ill elderly being cared for at home.
- *Rehabilitation centers.* The realization that an improved functional status will add quality to an impaired older person's life and be cost effective has launched geriatric rehabilitation as growing specialty.
- *Mental health centers.* Depressions and dementias are major problems affecting the older population, and recent advances in problem identification and therapeutic approaches have increased the elderly's use of outpatient psychiatric services to address these and other problems.
- *Day care, day treatment.* A variety of community-based programs have been developed as alternatives to institutionalization.
- *Sheltered housing, life care, retirement centers.* New forms of health services are emerging in response to the changing needs and life-styles of a new generation of older adults.

Even if nurses are in specialties that focus on the care of younger individuals, such as maternal and child health, they may still confront geriatric care issues as they work with families who have aged relatives. Thus it is the rare nurse who is not affected by or able to impact gerontologic care issues.

ROLES OF GERONTOLOGIC NURSES

One of the most exciting aspects of gerontologic nursing is the ability to use a wide range of knowledge and skills in delivering services, such as medical-surgical, psychiatric, and community health nursing; pharmacology; nutrition; thanatology; sociology; and psychology. This background is necessary to fulfill the diverse roles in geronotologic nursing, which are described following.

Teacher
Healthy aging starts early in life and so does education on practices to facilitate this process. The gerontologic nurse teaches persons of all ages the principles of good hygiene, nutrition, exercise, rest, stress management, and prevention of illness and injury. With the high prevalence of chronic illness among the elderly, nurses instruct clients in the management of conditions, including education concerning special diets, safe medication use, and treatment techniques. Also, gerontologic nurses educate other health care workers in new theory and practice related to the care of the elderly.

Counselor
Aging persons and their families face issues and decisions for which they have had little preparation, such as retirement, selecting a nursing home, caring for a sick spouse at home, widowhood, and grandparenting. The nurse can serve as a catalyst in helping individuals manage these situations by providing information, raising issues for consideration, guiding discussions, and linking with resources. In this way the nurse strengthens clients' abilities to deal with problems independently.

Care Giver
Many times, people cannot do things for themselves and require nursing services to partially or totally assist them. However, "doing for" older persons is not always necessary and often is not therapeutic. When an illness or disability exists and persons are unable to care for themselves independently, nurses need to first evaluate the barriers to self-care, which could include lack of knowledge or skills in care techniques; physical, emotional, or socioeconomic limitations; beliefs and attitudes; environmental obstacles; or poor motivation. Nursing actions should address the elimination or minimization of those barriers. Only when people are truly incapable of self-care (e.g., unconscious, severely demented, in need of special treatment) should nurses assume the function of completing actions for individuals.

Manager

In addition to the traditional managerial roles (e.g., charge nurse, supervisor) that nurses fill, gerontologic nurses can carve out creative roles as case managers in helping elderly persons access and coordinate services.

Advocate

Advocacy takes many forms in gerontologic nursing. For the individual client the nurse must ensure that the client's personal preferences and needs are respected and that the client is able to play an active role in decision making and the care process. For the elderly as a group, the nurse can support and recommend policies and programs that address needs in an ethical and practical way. This may be particularly important in the current economic climate to ensure that cost-saving measures do not threaten the provision of needed, high-quality services. For the specialty, the nurse needs to promote the status and practice of gerontologic nursing.

Specific situations may find nurses filling additional roles as subspecialization grows in gerontologic nursing (Box 1-2). Regardless of the position held, the gerontologic nurse's ultimate

---

BOX 1-2   Subspecialties in Gerontologic Nursing

Geropsychiatry
Rehabilitation
Nursing administration in long-term care, geriatric care settings
Chronic care
Case management
Critical care
Cardiac care
Trauma care
Surgical care
Cosmetic surgery counseling and care
Family care, family therapy
Sex therapy
Leisure health
Retirement health
Hospice
Health/patient education
Legal/ethical education

goal is to promote the highest level of health, function, and well-being in aging persons.

The challenge for gerontologic nurses in the future will be to continue the advancement of the specialty, prepare and recruit more nurses into this practice area, discover and implement new knowledge and skills, and improve the competency of all care givers who work with the elderly.

REFERENCES

Bishop LF: Relation of old age to disease with illustrative cases, *Am J Nurs* 4(4):674, 1904.
Nascher I: *Geriatrics,* Philadelphia, 1914, Blakiston.

2

❖ An Overview of Aging

FACTS ABOUT THE AGING POPULATION

Ours is an aging society both in the growing number of elderly people comprising it and the older median age for the entire population. At the end of the eighteenth century the median age was 16 years; it now exceeds 30 years, and by the year 2000 it will be 35 years. Just 4% of the population was 65 years of age or older at the beginning of the twentieth century; now the portion of elderly exceeds 12% and will reach 20% by the year 2030. American life expectancy is increasing although differences between the sexes and races exist (Table 2-1). White elders outnumber their cohorts of other races by 10:1, but this ratio will decrease as improved longevity among nonwhite groups, lower birth rates among whites, and immigration increase the proportion of other races in U.S. society.

An obvious outcome of life expectancy differences among the elderly is that women outnumber men in later years; there are approximately 7 older men for every 10 older women. The differences in life expectancy and the tendency for men to marry women younger than themselves (more than one third of men over 65 years of age have wives under 65 years of age) account for the fact that most older men have living spouses, whereas most older women are widowed. There are five widows for every widower in old age.

Not only are more people reaching old age than ever before, but they are living longer after they reach their sixty-fifth birthday than did earlier generations (Table 2-2). Thus the elderly population is becoming an older age group.

TABLE 2-1   U.S. Life Expectancies

	Male (yr)	Female (yr)
White	72.3	78.9
Nonwhite	64.9	73.4

From US Department of Commerce: *Statistical abstract of the United States,* ed 110, Washington, DC, 1990, Bureau of the Census, p 72.

TABLE 2-2   Increases in Survival of Aged to Old-Old Years

Year	Older population (%)		
	65-74 yr	75-84 yr	85 + yr
1900	71	25	4
1950	68	27	5
1975	62	30	8
2000 (est.)	55	34	11

From US Department of Commerce: *Statistical abstract of the United States,* ed 110, Washington, DC, 1990, Bureau of the Census, p 16.

Health and the Aged

Nearly 90% of all older people have a chronic illness. Chronic conditions are greater than four times more prevalent in the elderly than in other age groups. More often than not the older individual has several chronic illnesses for which medications and treatments must be juggled. Almost one half of the elderly have illnesses that interfere to some degree with their ability to engage in activities of daily living. The major chronic illnesses of the elderly, in order of prevalence, are as follows (U.S. Department of Commerce, 1990):

- Arthritis
- Hypertension
- Hearing impairments
- Heart conditions
- Chronic sinusitis
- Visual impairments
- Orthopedic problems
- Diabetes
- Varicose veins
- Hemorrhoids

BOX 2-1   Nine Leading Causes of Death for Population 65 Years and Over

Heart disease
Malignant neoplasms
Cerebrovascular disease
Chronic obstructive pulmonary disease
Pneumonia/influenza
Diabetes mellitus
Accidents and adverse effects
Chronic liver disease, cirrhosis
Suicide

From US Department of Commerce: *Statistical abstract of the United States*, ed 110, Washington, DC, 1990, Bureau of the Census, p 49.

Although acute conditions occur less frequently in later life, they are not insignificant. The elderly experience higher rates of complications and mortality from acute illnesses.

The leading causes of death for persons 65 years old and older are *heart disease, cancer,* and *stroke.* A review of the leading causes of death (Box 2-1) shows that accidents are a major threat to older persons. Sensorineural deficits and the effects of illnesses predispose the elderly to accidental injury. Although automobile-related accidents are the most common cause of accidental death in the 65- to 74-year-old group, falls rank first as the most common fatal injury for the entire older population.

Finances
In general, the elderly do not engage in a significant amount of preventive health care and screening. This may be due in part to the lack of insurance coverage for these practices.

Health care providers are in a cost-containment era and need to control costs of the insurance programs on which the elderly depend. Medicare pays the cost of most hospital care of older adults (Table 2-3); most of the Medicaid budget goes toward the cost of long-term care. Increasingly, questions are being raised about the disproportionate amount of public dollars spent on the 12% of the population who are aged and the ability of the system to continue to bear this expense as growing numbers of people reach old age.

Despite the amount of government benefits afforded the

TABLE 2-3   Sources of Reimbursement for Hospital Care of Elderly

Source	Percent of all sources
Medicare	93.4
Private insurance	4.1
Medicaid	0.9
Workers' compensation	0.7
Self-pay	0.5
Other	0.2

From US Department of Commerce: *Statistical abstract of the United States,* ed 110, Washington, DC, 1990, Bureau of the Census, p 111.

elderly, the financial status of most older adults is far from comfortable (Table 2-4). Social Security benefits, intended as a supplement to other sources of income, are the primary means of support for many elders. Just a minority of older adults receive private pension benefits; in fact, only approximately one half of all current workers are enrolled in pension plans to assist them in their old age. Few elderly are employed, constituting only a very small percent of the total labor force. Although the median net worth of the elderly is nearly twice that of other age groups (primarily because of the appreciated value of their homes), many elders find themselves cash poor to meet their ongoing financial demands. The fourth-ranking means of support for the elderly is public assistance. Many elderly recipients of public assistance depend on this means of support for the first time in their old age; they often become poor when they become old.

Home and Family
Very few individuals relocate to retirement communities or other locations in old age, most remain instead in the areas in which

TABLE 2-4   Annual Median Income of Older Individuals

	In dollars
Men	12,471
Women	7,103

From US Department of Commerce: *Statistical abstract of the United States,* ed 110, Washington, DC, 1990, Bureau of the Census, p 460.

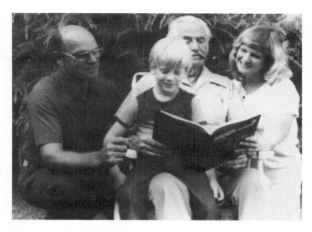

FIGURE 2-1 Most elderly have strong ties with their families. (From Castillo HM: *The nurse assistant in long-term care: a rehabilitative approach,* St Louis, 1992, Mosby–Year Book.)

they have lived most of their lives and, for the most part, in their same homes. Compared to other age groups, there is a higher proportion of old people in rural areas.

Most elderly have strong ties with their families (Figure 2-1). Less than one third have no families or live alone. Important assistance and support are exchanged between the elderly and their children. Although they have strong bonds, most elderly and their children prefer to live separately. Relationships between older spouses and siblings tend to strengthen and stabilize in late life.

THEORIES OF AGING

For centuries people have been interested in explaining why and how human beings age. Although this mystery has yet to be solved, several theories have attempted to explain the aging process (Box 2-2). They can be categorized as either *biologic* theories, which address the anatomic and physiologic changes occurring with age, or *psychosocial* theories, which explain the thought processes and behaviors of aging persons.

Theories of aging are hypotheses, not facts; no known single factor is responsible for the aging process. Aging is unique to each

BOX 2-2   Theories of Aging

BIOLOGIC

Free radical structure

Parts of molecules break off or the loose electrons from these free parts attach to other molecules causing altered cellular structure.

Environmental pollutants are believed to promote free radical activity.

Some foods especially thought to reduce free radical activity are those rich in vitamins A, C, and E.

Cross link of collagen

Collagen constitutes 25% to 30% of body protein and forms gelatin-like cell matrix. With age, collagen cross-links, becoming more insoluble and rigid.

Some chemicals are thought to reduce cross linkage (e.g., lathyrogens, prednisolone, and penicillamine).

Programmed cells

Just as the body possesses an inherited biologic clock that triggers events such as the onset of puberty, cells are believed to be programmed to "age" at specific times.

Autoimmune reactions

Immunologic system loses capacity for self-regulation and begins perceiving normal or age-altered cells as foreign matter. The system reacts by forming antibodies to destroy those cells.

A decline in the immunologic system is thought to allow the development of infections and cancer and to play a role in the development of diseases such as diabetes mellitus, atherosclerosis, hypertension, and rheumatic heart disease.

Lipofuscin

Lipofuscin is a lipoprotein by-product of metabolism, not known to have any function in the body. With age, lipofuscin accumulates, particularly in the liver, heart, ovaries, and neurons.

A relationship exists between age and the amount of accumulated lypofuscin.

Other species have been found to accumulate lipofuscin.

Somatic mutation

Such factors as DNA alteration, RNA mutation(s), and protein or enzyme synthesis cause defective cellular structure and function.

With age, defective cells multiply and lead to organ abnormalities, system dysfunction.

Continued.

BOX 2-2   Theories of Aging—cont'd

Stress

Repeated wear and tear impairs the efficiency of cellular function and eventually leads to physical decline.

Radiation

Laboratory studies reveal shorter life spans in rats, mice, and dogs exposed to nonlethal radiation doses; it is thought that the same can occur in humans. This theory is supported by the fact that ultraviolet light is known to cause solar elastosis (wrinkling of skin caused by replacement of collagen by elastin) and promote skin cancer.

Nutrition

The quality and quantity of diet is thought to influence life span.

   Problems caused by obesity, cholesterol, and vitamin deficiencies support this theory.

PSYCHOSOCIAL

Disengagement

Developed in late 1950s by Elaine Cummings and William Henry.

   Aging individuals and society gradually withdraw from each other for mutual benefit: societal activities can be transferred from old to young in orderly fashion, and older persons are allowed time to focus on self with reduced social burdens.

   Theory's popularity is undermined by the recognition that (1) each individual has a different aging pattern and (2) the process often damages both society and the aged.

Activity

Developed by Robert Havighurst in 1960s.

   Aging individuals should be expected to maintain norms of middle-aged adults: employment, activity, replacement of lost relationships.

   Age-related physical, mental, and socioeconomic losses may present legitimate obstacles to maintaining activity, thereby reducing universality of theory.

Development (continuity)

Described by Bernice Neugarten in 1960s; longitudinal studies still being conducted.

   Basic personality, attitude, and behaviors remain constant throughout the life span.

   Allows multiple options for aging and recognizes the individuality of the aging process.

individual. Certain factors can interfere with healthy aging, such as poor nutrition, excessive exposure to ultraviolet light, pollution, inadequate stress management, and disease-producing organisms. Factors that can promote healthy aging include a well-balanced diet, mental and physical activity, early detection and correction of health problems, and good hygiene.

Nursing Implications

If the theories of aging do nothing else, they should help nurses understand the variety of factors that impact the aging process. This results in a unique style of aging in each individual. Just as differences exist between 5-year-olds or 15-year-olds or 25-year-olds, no two 65-, 75-, or 85-year-olds will be identical either. In fact, with the many years of living they have experienced, elderly persons will probably show greater diversity than persons in other age groups. Astute assessment is needed to recognize the unique characteristics of the older client, and truly individualized care planning and delivery are crucial.

It is important to understand that nothing will eliminate or reverse the aging process. Immortality and eternal youth are not achievable. However, aging individuals can take actions to optimize a healthy aging process:

- Eating a nutritious diet in which calories and fats are controlled
- Limiting exposure to ultraviolet light
- Avoiding insults to the body, such as tobacco, drugs, and excessive noise
- Managing stress effectively
- Preventing infections and diseases, and identifying and treating them early if they do occur
- Maintaining a physically and mentally active state

DEVELOPMENTAL TASKS

Each stage of life possesses challenges, needs, and adjustments, known as developmental tasks. These tasks are part of an adult's continued growth through the life span. Successfully completed, these developmental tasks can bring satisfaction and a sense of psychosocial well-being in late life; unresolved, these tasks can cause unhappiness and bitterness about the life one has lived.

Various theorists have described the developmental tasks of late life, such as Erik Erikson (1959), Robert Peck (1968), Robert

BOX 2-3   Summary of Major Theorists' Views on the Developmental Tasks of Aging

Erikson believes that individuals face stages of psychologic development as they age:
- Trust vs. mistrust
- Autonomy vs. shame
- Initiative vs. guilt
- Industry vs. inferiority
- Identity vs. confusion
- Intimacy vs. isolation
- Generativity vs. stagnation
- Ego integrity vs. despair

The last stage, viewed as the major task in old age, is to accept one's life as having been whole and satisfying in order to achieve ego integrity. Dissatisfaction and regrets with the life one has lived can lead to a sense of despair and disgust.

Peck identifies three tasks faced in old age:
- *Ego differentiation vs. work-role preoccupation:* To develop satisfactions from one's self as a person rather than through the work role
- *Body transcendence vs. body preoccupation:* To find psychologic pleasures rather than becoming absorbed with the health problems or physical limitations imposed by aging
- *Ego transcendence vs. ego preoccupation:* To feel pleasure through reflecting on one's life rather than dwelling on the limited number of years left to live

Havighurst describes tasks of aging individuals to include the following:
- Adjusting to decreased strength and health status
- Maintaining involvement with friends and society
- Establishing satisfactory living arrangements
- Readjusting one's life-style to reduced income and retirement
- Coping with the death of one's spouse

Ebersole categorizes the developmental tasks of late life into three groups:
- *Receptive tasks:* Power and capacity in physical, social, cultural, and intellectual realms are relinquished and a certain amount of dependency is accepted
- *Expressive tasks:* A self-transcending philosophy is developed as older persons gain an appreciation for their place in life and the legacy they leave
- *Dynamic tasks:* These tasks entail not only one's own physical and psychologic dying process but also helping others learn about death

Butler and **Lewis** view the major tasks of late life as follows:
- Adjusting to one's infirmities
- Developing a sense of satisfaction with the life that has been lived
- Preparing for death

Modified from Eliopoulos C: Developmental tasks of aging, *Long-Term Care Educator* 2(lesson 6):4, 1991.

Havighurst (1974), Priscilla Ebersole (1976), and Robert Butler and Myrna Lewis (1982). Box 2-3 summarizes these theories. The common themes throughout each of the various theories of developmental tasks of aging are that the elderly must adjust to significant changes, find meaning in their existence, and prepare for death.

Nurses must appreciate that many older adults face developmental tasks at a time when physical, emotional, and social reserves are reduced. Nursing assistance may be required to enable the elderly to face these challenges; this can be achieved by the following actions:

- Helping clients maintain and establish roles and relationships
- Offering maximum opportunities for decision making
- Learning about and building on clients' unique interests and skills
- Listening to clients' concerns
- Asking clients about and encouraging discussions of past accomplishments and experiences
- Introducing activities that can promote reminiscence

Nursing staff should not underestimate the significance of their own attitudes toward aging. Staff who view aging as a process of continuous decline and old age as a depressing, useless period may treat the elderly as though they are hopeless and helpless. Conversely, staff who believe that every stage of life brings new opportunities and challenges may approach older persons with encouragement and optimism. A self-examination of their own attitudes and clarification of values may be necessary for staff members who work with the elderly.

PHYSICAL CHANGES WITH AGE

With age the number of cells gradually declines, so that by the time an individual reaches age 70 there are 30% fewer functioning cells in the body. Obviously, a 30% shrinkage in the size of the body does not occur, so a compensatory mechanism must exist. The cells enlarge in size, so that fewer but larger cells make up the body, making its total mass appear relatively unaltered. Also, aged cells are of irregular structure. The many alterations in organ function result from these basic changes on the cellular level.

The fluid within the cell decreases although extracellular fluid and plasma volume remain constant. The reduction in intracellular fluid results in less total body fluid, which is one of the major reasons for dehydration occurring more easily in older persons.

Tissues are lost throughout the body, with the exception of adipose tissue. A higher proportion of the body's composition is fat, a consideration in the nutritional assessment and prescription of drugs (many drugs are stored in adipose tissue). The loss of subcutaneous tissue is evidenced through a deepening of the hollows of intercostal and supraclavicular spaces, orbits, and axillae and sagging breasts. Reduced subcutaneous tissue causes less natural insulation and a more severe response to temperature fluctuation.

Some of the other general changes in body composition include a progressive decrease in serum albumin, an increase in globulin, a slow increase in serum cholesterol throughout adulthood with a stabilization or slight decrease after the sixth decade, decreased ability to metabolize glucose, and higher blood glucose levels in the absence of diabetes.

Cardiovascular

Normally, the size of the heart does not change with age, however, the valves become thick and rigid because of sclerosis and fibrosis. As a compensatory measure for less efficient oxygen use, the aortic volume and systolic blood pressure rise.

Decreased efficiency of the heart muscle reduces cardiac output by approximately 1% per year during adulthood. Although this does not significantly affect the resting heart rate, profound effects are noted under stressful or unusual conditions: the heart will take longer (sometimes several hours) to return to its normal rate. There is greater peripheral resistance in vessels caused by calcium deposits, cross linking of collagen, and a reduction in elastin. Capillary walls are thicker, which may impede the effective exchange of nutrients and promote capillary fragility.

Pulmonary

The lungs lose elasticity and become more rigid with age. This results in an increased residual capacity, a lower vital capacity, decreased maximum breathing capacity, and a greater likelihood of collapse during opening of the chest cavity or pneumothorax.

Alveoli are fewer in number and larger in size. Alveolar ducts and bronchioles have an increased diameter. There is less ciliary activity. The anteroposterior chest diameter increases. As a result, the thoracic transverse measurement may be reduced. Costal cartilage calcification and partial contraction of the inspiratory muscles cause decreased mobility of the ribs. Weaker thoracic inspiratory and expiratory muscles create conditions that promote respiratory infections, including incomplete lung expansion, insufficient basilar inflation, decreased ability to expel foreign or accumulated material, and inefficient cough response.

Blood oxygen level (Po_2) decreases by 10% to 15%. Although blood carbon dioxide level (Pco_2) remains constant, the high prevalence in the elderly of chronic obstructive lung disease, which raises Pco_2 levels, frequently causes elevated levels. Oxygen use under stress is reduced because of delayed oxygen diffusion, ineffective perfusion, and inefficient use of oxygen by stressed tissues.

Gastrointestinal
Teeth are not usually lost as a result of normal aging although a history of poor dental health and dietary practices has caused more than 50% of today's elderly to be edentulous (Figure 2-2). Periodontal disease becomes the number one cause of tooth loss after 30 years of age. If natural teeth exist they tend to have flatter surfaces, stains, and varying degrees of erosion and abrasion of

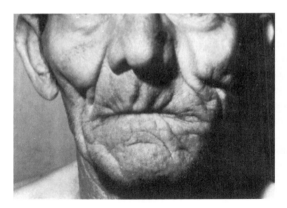

FIGURE 2-2 Face of old person with typical age changes. (From Papas AS, Niessen LC, Chauncey HH: *Geriatric dentistry: aging and oral health,* St Louis, 1991, Mosby–Year Book.)

the crown and root structure. Teeth that are loose or break easily can be aspirated, creating the risk of lung infections and abscesses.

Approximately one third the volume of saliva produced in youth is produced in old age; thus the mixing and swallowing of food, tablets, and capsules can be difficult without ample fluid intake. The decreased secretion of salivary ptyalin interferes with the digestion of starch. Atrophy of the epithelial covering occurs in the oral mucosa.

In late life approximately one third the number of taste buds per papilla remain, which causes the taste threshold to increase. Pipe smoking causes a more profound loss. The receptors for sweet and salty flavors are affected most, and food distastes can result.

Aspiration of food becomes a greater risk because of a weaker gag reflex, delayed emptying of the esophagus as a result of its slight dilation and decreased peristalsis, relaxation of the lower esophageal sphincter, and reduced stomach motility and emptying. Smaller volumes of food should be consumed at each meal, and the individual should remain upright during and approximately 30 minutes after meals.

Hunger contractions are reduced because of less motor activity in the stomach. In addition, within the stomach the mucosal lining is thinner, digestive juice (hydrochloric acid, pepsin, pancreatic enzymes) production is reduced, and fats are less well tolerated, which is believed to be associated with decreased lipase production.

Some atrophy occurs along the small and large intestines. The internal anal sphincter is believed to lose its tone although research in this area is inconclusive at present. The elderly are predisposed to constipation as a result of decreased colonic peristalsis and slower and duller neural impulses, which dull the signal to defecate.

The liver decreases in weight and storage capacity. Gallstone incidence increases because of less efficient cholesterol stabilization and absorption. Although the levels remain adequate for digestive functions, there is a reduction in the volume and concentration of pancreatic enzymes. The pancreas gains more fat content.

Genitourinary

Decreased tissue growth, a loss of nephrons, and atherosclerosis cause the renal mass to become smaller with age. The function of the kidneys is altered by a reduction in the glomerular filtration rate (nearly 50% between youth and old age), a 50% decrease in renal blood flow resulting from a lower filtration rate, and a decline in tubular function causing less effective concentration of urine and a decreased reabsorption of glucose from the filtrate. These changes create problems such as delayed filtration of drugs from the bloodstream and unreliability of urine testing for glucose.

Decreased bladder capacity and a delayed micturition reflex create problems for the elderly in urinary frequency, urgency, and nocturia. Urinary retention is more prevalent among the elderly. Incontinence is not a normal outcome of aging although many postmenopausal women (particularly those who had several pregnancies) experience stress incontinence caused by a weakening of the pelvic diaphragm.

A majority of older men have some degree of prostatic enlargement, which increases urinary frequency. Most of this hypertrophy is benign, but it produces a greater risk of malignancy. Thus regular evaluation is essential.

Male reproductive system changes include the following:
- Decreased testosterone production
- Reduced sperm count
- Smaller testes
- Lower viscosity of seminal fluid
- Need for more direct physical stimulation to achieve an erection
- Lengthened time needed to regain erection after interruption or completed intercourse

Female reproductive system changes include the following:
- Decreased estrogen production
- Reduction in breast tissue
- Shrinkage of uterus
- More alkaline vaginal secretions, increasing the risk of vaginitis
- Narrowing, shortening, and increased fragility of vaginal canal
- Drier vaginal canal, necessitating longer foreplay or use of lubricant to facilitate penile penetration

There is no change in libido in either sex. The common age-related changes do not prohibit sexual expression in older persons. Patterns of sexual activity and preference tend to be consistent throughout the life span.

Musculoskeletal

The muscles experience a loss of cells, overall mass, strength, and movement. Muscle tremors often occur, believed to be associated with degeneration of the extrapyramidal system. Bones become brittle and easy to fracture, as a result of a gradual resorption of the interior surface of long bones and slower new bone production on the outside surface. The cartilage surface of joints deteriorates, which limits joint activity and range of motion. Between 20 and 70 years of age, there is approximately a 2-inch reduction in height due to thinner intervertebral disks, shortening of the vertebral column associated with cartilage loss, and slight kyphosis and flexion of the hips and knees.

Neurologic

Nerve cells are lost with age, and nerve conduction velocity decreases. The response to multiple stimuli and kinesthetic sense is reduced. Most reflexes are slowed although deep tendon reflexes are retained. Stages 3 and 4 of sleep become less prominent. It is not unusual for sleep to be frequently interrupted; however, the actual amount of sleep loss is minimal.

Sensory

The effects of aging on vision are profound, including the following:

- Presbyopia, a farsightedness that begins in the fourth decade of life and causes most older people to require corrective lenses
- Narrowing of the visual field
- Smaller pupil size, reducing visual adaptation to darkness
- Yellowing of the lens, distorting low-tone colors such as blues, greens, and violets
- Opacity of the lens, causing glare to be a greater problem
- Less efficient resorption of intraocular fluid, increasing the risk of glaucoma
- Distorted depth perception
- Development of arcus senilis (a partial or complete glossy white circle around the periphery of the iris)
- Reduced lacrimal secretions, allowing eyes to become irritated more easily

Hearing also undergoes serious changes that can threaten the elderly's maintenance of a safe and normal life-style. *Presbycusis* is the term used to describe age-related hearing loss that involves a dysfunction in the ability to transmit nerve impulses from the ear to the brain. Initially, high-frequency sounds (e.g., s, sh, ph, f, and ch) are filtered from the speech; as the condition progresses, middle and low frequencies are impacted. Hearing can be mechanically blocked by cerumen, which contains more keratin (making it of a harder consistency) and accumulates, forming an impaction.

The threshold for pain and touch increases. Conditions causing severe pain in younger persons can cause only minor pain or a sense of pressure in the elderly. The reduced ability to feel pressure increases the risk of skin breakdown. Alterations in proprioception (sense of physical position) can cause problems with balance and spatial orientation.

Olfaction is diminished, reducing the ability to identify hazards in the environment and to enjoy the pleasurable scents of the environment.

Integumentary
With age the skin becomes less elastic, drier, and more fragile, demonstrated by wrinkling and sagging. The risk of skin breakdown increases. "Age spots" or "liver spots" develop as a result of clustering of melanocytes; this excessive pigmentation most often occurs in areas of the body exposed to the sun. Scalp, pubic, and axilla hair thins and loses color, whereas hair in the nose and ears thickens. Women may find that they develop some facial hair. Fingernails grow at a slower rate and become thick and brittle.

Endocrine
The pituitary gland loses weight and vascularity and contains increased amounts of connective tissue. Although follicle-stimulating hormone (FSH) increases in women, adrenocorticotropic hormone (ACTH), antidiuretic hormone (ADH), thyroid-stimulating hormone (TSH), luteinizing hormone (LH), growth hormone (GH), and male FSH do not change.

A variety of changes impact the thyroid gland. Fibrosis, cellular infiltration, and increased modularity occur. A decrease in plasma T_3 is seen, as well as a reduction in radioiodine accumulation and a lower basal metabolic rate. Plasma T_4 is unchanged.

Insulin release by the beta cells of the pancreas is delayed. Some reduced peripheral sensitivity to circulating insulin is also thought to occur. Increased blood glucose levels in nondiabetic older persons are not uncommon and necessitate the use of age-related gradients for interpreting glucose tolerance tests.

The adrenal glands in old age are characterized by increased amounts of connective tissue, reduced lipid, pigmentation, cortical nodules, and reductions in secretion of cortisol; the plasma level of ACTH is normal. Blood level and urinary excretion of aldosterone, adrenal androgen production, and epinephrine and norepinephrine (although research supporting this is inconclusive at this point) are increased also.

Ovarian-produced estrogen ceases after menopause; there is no significant change in adrenal-produced estrogen. Progesterone production and excretion are decreased. Testosterone production and metabolic clearance rates decline. Less parathyroid hormone (PTH) is secreted by the parathyroid gland.

PSYCHOLOGIC/COGNITIVE CHANGES

Personality

There is no stereotypic profile of an older person. People do not become wise, feeble, childlike, rigid, or cantankerous in old age. Their basic psychologic characteristics will remain with them throughout their lives, resulting in diversity in psychologic status in advanced age. Personality changes in old age can be associated with physical or mental health problems.

Intelligence

Basic intelligence is maintained. The wise old person most likely was bright when young, while mentally dull elderly may never have had a high IQ. Crystallized intelligence, which enables the person to rely on past learning and experiences for problem solving, is usually maintained or grows slowly throughout the life span. Fluid intelligence, which controls emotions, retention of nonintellectual information, creative capacities, spatial perceptions, and esthetic appreciation, shows some decline in late life. With increasing age, more time is needed to solve problems. Significant changes in intelligence usually are associated with physical or mental health problems.

IQ test performance of older adults may be hindered because of sensory deficits or the stress of being tested. These factors must be considered when assessing intelligence.

Memory

Long-term memory for information not used on a daily basis can be slowed with age. The decline in short-term memory, long believed to be a normal outcome of aging, is now considered to be more related to a lack of use of this function than a normal consequence of aging; the use of memory aids (mnemonic devices) can improve some age-related memory problems. Poor health status can threaten both long- and short-term memory.

Learning
Past learning experiences and attitudes affect learning capacity in old age, as does the presence of health problems. Older adults may tend to rely more on previous solutions to problems rather than experiment with new problem-solving techniques. The early learning phase is more difficult and longer for older adults; however, after a longer early phase the elderly are able to keep pace with younger learners. Older persons show some difficulty with perceptual motor tasks.

Attention Span
Older adults are more easily distracted by stimuli, are less able to retain information longer than 45 minutes (decreased vigilance performance), and have more difficulty performing tasks that are complicated or that require simultaneous performance.

Normal aging does not cause disorientation, loss of language or calculation abilities, poor judgment, or any other type of mental dysfunction. Signs of poor cognitive function signal a physical or mental health problem and warrant a thorough evaluation.

REFERENCES

Butler RN, Lewis MI: *Aging and mental health,* ed 3, St Louis, 1982, Mosby–Year Book.

Ebersole P: Developmental tasks in later life. In Burnside I, editor: *Nursing and the aged,* New York, 1976, McGraw-Hill.

Erikson E: *Childhood and society,* ed 2, New York, 1959, Norton.

Havighurst R: *Developmental tasks and education,* ed 3, New York, 1974, David McKay.

Peck R: Psychological developments in the second half of life. In Neugarten B, editor: *Middle age and aging,* Chicago, 1968, University of Chicago Press.

US Department of Commerce: *Statistical abstract of the United States,* ed 110, Washington, DC, 1990, Bureau of the Census, p 118.

3

The Nursing Process and the Elderly

Many of the health care needs presented by older adults can be appropriately identified and managed by nurses. The fact that nursing personnel are the major source of workers in geriatric care settings attests to the significant role of nursing. Professional nursing meets this challenge by offering services in a planned, organized, and individualized manner rather than approaching care needs in a fragmented way or solely through the fulfillment of medical orders. This systematic approach to nursing care is called the *nursing process* and consists of four general components: assessment, diagnosis and planning, implementation, and evaluation.

ASSESSMENT

Assessment is the process of collecting and analyzing data. This is an ongoing activity because it occurs with every nurse-client encounter. Every time a nurse communicates with clients, administers medications, performs a treatment, or observes clients in activities, physical status and mental status are evaluated. The continuous nature of the assessment process provides a comprehensive picture of clients and is more likely to identify changes in status than a one-time snapshot obtained through a formal intake/admission assessment. Box 3-1 outlines some of the data reviewed during the assessment and possible findings.

The quantity and quality of data collected depends on the

Text continued on p. 39.

BOX 3-1   Guidelines for Assessing Older Adults

GENERAL INFORMATION
Name
Date of birth
Address
Telephone
Contact person
Educational level
Financial status
Occupational history
Religion
Languages spoken
Advance directive

Although the collection of general demographic data seems quite straight-forward, the process used to obtain this information can yield significant insight into the client's cognitive abilities. Memory deficits can be apparent with the client's inability to recall address or telephone number. Ask the date of birth to aid in assessing long-term memory; follow this with the question, "So how old did that make you on your last birthday?" to further assess mental status.

When asking about address, review the housing circumstances of the client, including ability to maintain and afford home, safety, security, proximity of shopping and services, and relationship with neighbors.

If it has not already been reviewed by a social worker, assess the client's financial status. This is done by listing all sources of income and all expenses and determining the difference between the two. A client with limited funds may be unable to comply with health or medical care recommendations, such as purchasing prescriptions, eating a special diet, and obtaining follow-up care. Ensure that the client is using all health and social services and benefits to which he or she is entitled. Occupational history not only yields information related to financial status, but also can provide insight into health conditions of the client. Review all major jobs held by the client with consideration of the occupational risks associated with those jobs and how these relate to the client's current health status. (For instance, respiratory problems in late life may be due to asbestos exposure in earlier years.) If the client is actively employed, ask the reason for employment: the client who reluctantly works in old age because he or she can not make ends meet otherwise differs from the one who works because of the satisfactions and challenges derived. If the client is retired, review adjustment to the retiree role.

Review the religion and religious practices of the client. If the client practices a religion with which staff members are unfamiliar, seek a resource person who can provide information and guidance to staff (e.g., regarding special practices, dietary restrictions, holy days). Ask the client for the name of the church, temple,or congregation in which he or she is active; this organization may be helpful in providing services to the client.

Continued.

BOX 3-1   Guidelines for Assessing Older Adults—cont'd

The client's fluency with the English language most likely will be obvious during the interview; however, it is beneficial to learn of other languages used by the client. It is not unusual for people to resort to native languages when feeling stressed; knowing that the client is bilingual can help staff members understand this situation if it should occur. An interpreter should be obtained for the client with limited ability to use the English language.

Determine if an advance directive exists and ensure that it is clearly communicated in the client's health record. If the client has not developed an advance directive, recommend that the physician or other appropriate resource person review this matter with the client.

FAMILY PROFILE
Marital status
Members
Roles, responsibilities
Support system
Pets

Ask about current marital status. If the spouse is living, review the spouse's age, health status, and functional ability. Determine if the spouse requires assistance and care from the client or vice versa. Whereas most older men have living spouses, most older women are widowed. Explore reactions to widowhood, resolution of grief, problems resulting from widowhood (e.g., reduced income, inability to maintain home, lack of social life).

Review location, relationship, ages, and health status of children. Most older adults have at least weekly contact with children and exchange assistance with them. Identify children or other family members who are willing and able to assist the client. (Keep in mind that family members play various roles in the family unit and may not share responsibilities equally.) Discuss the client's wishes concerning having the care plan and care activities shared with family members.

Increasing numbers of families are providing complicated, continuous care for older persons for a long period of time; cost containment efforts could increase care-giving burdens of families. Ask about care-giving activities and resources used. Determine the impact of care giving on the care giver or care givers and the entire family unit. Arrange for training, respite, and related services as needed.

Review nonrelated "significant others" who share a special relationship with the client and who may be included in the client's care activities.

Pets are important members of many families and can be particularly important to older adults. Ask about pets and the ability to care for them. Since some clients may be reluctant to be hospitalized or have other extended periods away from home because of concern about the care of their pets, assist clients in arranging pet care if necessary. Be aware that the loss of a pet can produce

BOX 3-1   Guidelines for Assessing Older Adults—cont'd

the same depression and grief reactions as the loss of any other loved one; this should be considered when determining the possible reasons for symptoms.

LIFE-STYLE
Activities
Social and leisure patterns
Typical day
Ask for a description of the client's typical day and how this compares with the lifelong activity pattern (e.g., usual time of awakening, meal pattern, naps, routines, bedtime). Review social and leisure activities enjoyed by the client. Keep in mind that most persons continue the same patterns of social and leisure activities in late life that they have enjoyed throughout their lives. Determine how health problems have affected life-style and the client's reaction.

HEALTH HISTORY
Self-evaluation of health
Health problems
Allergies
Health practices
Health goals
The correlation between perceived and real health status can yield insights regarding acceptance of diagnoses, educational needs, mental status, and coping skills. Ask the client to describe health conditions he/she is aware of possessing and the practices followed to manage those conditions. Discuss the client's views of his/her own health status (e.g., how he thinks he compares to other people his age, how he would rate his health on a scale from 1 to 10).

Ask the client to describe any symptoms or signs. Offer specifics to trigger the client's memory (e.g., "Do you have any shortness of breath, pain, indigestion, dizziness, blackouts?").

Review health practices of the client, such as diet, exercise, use of vitamins, meditation, and unconventional practices. Ask about the use of alcohol and drugs. The poor memory of many older clients and the stress of being interviewed can cause some clients to forget allergies. Review specific substances and describe specific allergic reactions to assist in triggering memory (e.g., "Have you ever developed a rash, hives, dizziness, vomiting, or confusion from any drug, chemical, plant, material, eggs or other food?"). Likewise, when reviewing previous illnesses and hospitalizations give specific items to which the client can react (e.g., "Have you ever had a broken bone, hysterectomy, heart attack, blood transfusion? Has any health professional ever told you that you have diabetes, heart disease, high blood pressure?")

Determine the dates of screening examinations and refer client if in need of an examination:

Continued.

BOX 3-1   Guidelines for Assessing Older Adults—cont'd

Test	Recommended Frequency
Mammogram	Annually
Breast examination	Annually
Pap smear	Every 1–3 years
Pelvic examination	Annually
Blood cholesterol	Every 3–5 years
Digital rectal examination	Annually
Prostate	Annually
Stool for occult blood	Annually
Sigmoidoscopy	Every 3–5 years
Urinalysis	Annually
Vision	Every 1–2 years
Hearing	Every 1–2 years

Ask the client to describe what he/she hopes to obtain from this hospitalization, home visit, office visit or nursing home stay. Determine motivation to participate in self-care activities, maintain or regain independence, and comply with the care plan as well as the client's understanding of the actual objective of the service provided.

MEDICATION HISTORY
Drugs used
Effects
Review all prescription and nonprescription drugs used by the client on a regular or an occasional basis. Determine the client's understanding of the appropriate use and purpose of each drug. Ask about the effectiveness of the drug and side effects. Check that the dosages have been adjusted for the client's age and health status, that the drugs continue to be needed, and that interactions are not a risk with the drugs used.

VITAL SIGNS
Temperature
Pulse
Respirations
Blood pressure
Obtain body temperature. Be aware that rectal and tympanic temperatures tend to register about 1°F higher than oral temperatures, whereas axillary temperatures usually are 1°F lower. Rectal temperatures do not respond tochanges in arterial temperatures as quickly as oral or tympanic temperatures, and inaccuracies in rectal temperature can occur if the thermometer is inserted at different sites within the rectum each time or there is stool in the rectum.

BOX 3-1 Guidelines for Assessing Older Adults—cont'd

Body temperature normally falls within a range between 96°F and 99°F. Impaired thermoregulation often occurs in old age and causes older adults to have lower normal body temperatures. The healthy baseline temperature for the individual client should be established and used to evaluate febrile conditions (e.g., a client with a normal temperature of 97°F has a fever when his or her temperature is 99°F). Also, the time of day in which the temperature is assessed is significant to note because temperature fluctuates during the day, being at its lowest in the early morning and peaking in the early evening.

Assess the apical and radial pulses; a difference in these pulses (pulse deficit) is abnormal. Note the rate, rhythm, and volume of the pulse. Since the older adult's heart can take several hours to return to its baseline norm after being stressed, a review of activities in the preceding hours is necessary when tachycardia is discovered.

The rate, rhythm, character, and depth of respirations should be assessed. Full, deep respirations, consistent with good aeration of the lungs, are noted by movement of the stomach during breathing. Auscultate the breath sounds and describe findings.

Assess blood pressure in three positions (lying, sitting, and standing); drops greater than 20 mm Hg in different positions are considered significant. Age-related changes to the cardiovascular system necessitate some increase in blood pressure to provide adequate circulation; however, caution is advised to ensure blood pressure is not excessively high to risk cerebrovascular accident and other complications. Usually, repeated elevations above 160 mm Hg systolic and 90 mm Hg diastolic are considered suspicious of hypertension; clients with these findings should be referred for further evaluation.

HEIGHT, WEIGHT
Obtain the client's height without shoes. Approximately 2 inches of height are lost between 20 and 70 years of age because of some loss of cartilage and thinning of the vertebrae.

Weigh the client, and use an age-adjusted scale to determine the appropriateness of the client's weight. (An age-adjusted scale recommends heavier normal weight ranges than the Metropolitan Life Insurance Company recommendations [Table 3-1].) Weight losses greater than 5% of body weight within the past month or 10% within the past 6 months are considered significant and should be evaluated further. Ask the client how current height and weight compare to those of earlier years.

SKIN STATUS
Color
Turgor
Moisture
Integrity

Continued on p. 36.

TABLE 3-1 Comparison of the Weight-for-Height Tables from Acturial Data (Build Study): Non-Age-Corrected Metropolitan Life Insurance Company and Age-Specific Gerontology Research Center Recommendations*

Height (ft-in)	Metropolitan 1983 weights (lb) for 25-59 yr†		Gerontology research center weight range for men and women (lb)‡					
	Men	Women	25 yr	35 yr	45 yr	55 yr	65 yr
4-10	—	100-131	84-111	92-119	99-127	107-135	115-142
4-11	—	101-134	87-115	95-123	103-131	111-139	119-147
5-0	—	103-137	90-119	98-127	106-135	114-143	123-152
5-1	123-145	93-123	101-131	110-140	118-148	127-157	
5-2	125-148	108-144	96-127	105-136	113-144	122-153	131-163
5-3	127-151	111-148	99-131	108-140	117-149	126-158	135-168
5-4	129-155	114-152	102-135	112-145	121-154	130-163	140-173
5-5	131-159	117-156	106-140	115-149	125-159	134-168	144-179
5-6	133-163	109-144	119-154	129-164	138-174	148-184	

Height							
5-7	135-167	123-164	112-148	122-159	133-169	143-179	153-190
5-8	137-171	126-167	116-153	126-163	137-174	147-184	158-196
5-9	139-175	129-170	119-157	130-168	141-179	151-190	162-201
5-10	141-179	132-173	122-162	134-173	145-184	156-195	167-207
5-11	144-183	135-176	126-167	137-178	149-190	160-201	172-213
6-0	147-187	—	129-171	141-183	153-195	165-207	177-219
6-1	150-192	—	133-176	145-188	157-200	169-213	182-225
6-2	153-197	—	137-181	149-194	162-206	174-219	187-232
6-3	157-202	—	141-186	153-199	166-212	179-225	192-238
6-4	—	—	144-191	157-205	171-218	184-231	197-244

*Values in this table are for height without shoes and weight without clothes. To convert inches to centimeters, multiply by 2.54; to convert pounds to kilograms, multiply by 0.455.

†The weight range is the lower weight for small frame and the upper weight for large frame.

‡Data from Andres R: Mortality and obesity; the rationale for age-specific height-weight tables. In Andres R, Bierman EL, Hazzard WR, editors: *Principles of geriatric medicine*, New York, 1985, McGraw-Hill, p 311.

From Andres R, Elalu D, Tobin JD et al: Impact of age on weight goals, *Ann Intern Med* 103(6):1032, 1985.

BOX 3-1   Guidelines for Assessing Older Adults—cont'd

Inspect the entire surface of the client's skin. It is best to conduct this inspection in a room with nonfluorescent lighting because fluorescent lights make it more difficult to detect minor rashes and lesions. Note discolorations and lesions, and describe their characteristics (e.g., measured diameter, color, location, type, configuration).

Decreased skin elasticity is a common finding in most older adults and can make the assessment of skin turgor more difficult. The areas of the body least affected by age-related decreases in elasticity are the skin over the forehead and sternum; these are the best places to evaluate skin turgor.

Use the back of the hand to make a gross evaluation of skin temperature. Note moisture of the skin. Compare findings bilaterally.

FUNCTIONAL STATUS
Activities of daily living (ADL)
Instrumental activities of daily living (IADL)

Evaluate the client's independence in ADLs, that is, bathing, dressing, toileting, moving, transferring, continence, and feeding. Observe the client's gait and note abnormalities and tolerance in ambulating distances.

Ask the client about independence in performing IADLs, that is, ability to use the telephone, shop, prepare meals, clean house, launder clothes, travel in the community, take medications, and manage money.

If the client lacks full independence in any of the ADLs or IADLs, describe the amount of independence that is possessed and the specific type of assistance required. Describe assistive aids used by the client. Discuss the client's reactions to deficits.

ORAL HEALTH

Tooth loss is not a normal outcome of aging; however, most of today's elderly lack a full set of natural teeth. Describe amount and condition of teeth. With a gloved hand, palpate and inspect the oral mucosa and tongue. Note lesions, friction rubs, discolorations, and other abnormalities. If dentures are worn, determine condition and fit; ask the client when the dentures were obtained (it is not unusual for dentures to fit poorly after approximately 5 years because of changes in tissue structure of gums and a faster rate of bone resorption in the absence of teeth).

Determine moisture of the oral cavity. Note odors and describe as specifically as possible; many odors are associated with pathologic conditions (e.g., urine odor to breath can occur with uremic acidosis; sweet, cloverlike odor can result from liver failure). Ask client about the ability to chew food and swallow. Describe abnormalities.

EATING PATTERN

Ask the client how and when he/she eats, the type and amount of food consumed, and recent changes in food intake. Review appetite. Discuss unique

BOX 3-1   Guidelines for Assessing Older Adults—cont'd

cultural, ethnic, or religious dietary preferences or restrictions. Question about food allergies or intolerances. Discuss the factors that could interfere with adequate dietary intake, such as limited finances, inability to cook, and social isolation. Review the amount and type of fluid intake per day.

ELIMINATION PATTERN
Ask about voiding pattern, continence, and symptoms of urinary problems (e.g., frequency, voiding, burning, urgency). If incontinence is present, ask about type, pattern, frequency of occurrence, and management.

Review pattern of bowel elimination, continence, and symptoms. Ask client about laxative and enema use. Unless contraindicated, perform digital rectal examination and test stool for blood. If hemorrhoids are present, review symptoms, management, and signs of blood loss.

SPEECH AND HEARING
Throughout the interview, determine the client's ability to understand and appropriately use language. Assess voice tone and quality, articulation, and speech pattern. Note aphasia (associated with neurologic disease or altered cognition) and monotonous or slurred speech (associated with neurologic disease, intoxication, hypoglycemia).

Inspect ears for cerumen accumulation and discharge. Ask about tinnitus, itching, pain. Determine client's ability to hear normal speech; hold a watch to client's ear and evaluate ability to hear ticking. Presbycusis, the sensorineural hearing loss associated with aging, is a common finding and frequently is noted by a difficulty hearing high-pitched sounds. Refer for audiometric evaluation if hearing has not been tested within past year or hearing problems are noted.

VISION
Presbyopia results in farsightedness and causes most older adults to wear corrective lenses. Determine visual acuity by having client read a Snellen chart or different-sized print headings from a newspaper; describe the size of print the client is able to see (e.g., can read small print with use of eyeglasses, cannot see print less than 1 inch in size). If client is unable to see any letters on newspaper, determine if client can see the number of fingers being held in front of face or if vision is so poor that he/she can only see people or objects as large dark figures.

Assess peripheral vision by sitting at eye level with the client, approximately 3 feet away, asking the client to look at your eyes, and stretching your arm with your index finger pointed; gradually bring your finger into the peripheral field and determine when the client is able to see your finger. Systematically test all points along a 360 degree area. With some conditions, such as cerebrovascular accident (CVA) and glaucoma, reductions in visual field are noted.

Ask client about problems with glare or vision that is hazy or unclear; positive

Continued.

BOX 3-1   Guidelines for Assessing Older Adults—cont'd

findings can be associated with cataracts. If client has had cataract removal, note if intraocular lens implant was used.

Review date of last ophthalmologic examination (including tonometry) and refer if testing has not been done within past year or if abnormal findings are present.

SLEEP AND REST PATTERN
Ask about usual time of going to bed and awakening, feeling on awakening (e.g., rested and refreshed or dull and fatigued), interruptions to sleep, use of sleep inducers, and number and length of naps. Normally, older adults need about 5 to 7 hours of sleep and one nap during the day. Review symptoms that may occur during the night, such as dyspnea, nightmares, confusion, urinary frequency, and muscle cramps.

SEXUAL HISTORY
Discuss client's satisfaction with recent changes in, and problems with sexual function. Normally, older adults should be able to engage in sex and achieve orgasm. Sexual dysfunction could be associated with a variety of factors, including side effects from medications, stress, depression, and medical problems.

MENTAL HEALTH
Mental health history
Symptoms
Cognition
Level of consciousness
Review client's history of treatment and hospitalization for mental health problems. (You may need to use questions such as, "Have you ever had a nervous breakdown? Did you ever need tranquilizers to help get you through a bad time? Did you ever need treatment for bad nerves or moodiness?")

Ask about symptoms related to mental health problems, such as sleep disorders, appetite changes, disinterest in activities, suspiciousness, hallucinations, delusions, inability to control actions, suicidal thoughts, euphoria, and extreme sadness.

Note mood and appropriateness of behavior.

Altered cognition can be associated with a variety of physical and mental disorders.

To assess cognition determine the following:
- *Orientation.* To person, place, and time
- *Retention and recall.* Ability to remember three unrelated words immediately and after 15 minutes
- *Judgment.* Ability to give reasonable response to a problem or situation that is presented (e.g., "What would you do if you saw something on fire in the trash can?")

BOX 3-1 Guidelines for Assessing Older Adults—cont'd

- *Three-stage command.* Ability to follow three related directions (e.g., pick up the paper, fold it in half, and give it to me)
- *Language competency.* Ability to state proper name of common object, construct sentence, speak coherently
- *Calculation.* Ability to count backward from 100 by 7s (must be able to successfully subtract five times, i.e., 100, 93, 86, 79, 72)

Normally, older adults should be able to perform all aspects of the cognitive test. Sometimes, the stress of being interviewed or going through an admission process may cause some older persons to perform poorly on the test. Rather than engraving results in stone, it is best to retest the client at a later time, after he/she has had a chance to relax and adjust.

Problems in cognition could be caused by acute (delirium) or chronic (dementia) disorders. On first contact, the client who has delirium may look similar to the client with dementia, because they both have impaired cognition. However, history of onset (rapid with delirium; slow and subtle with dementia) and level of consciousness (altered with delirium; unchanged with dementia) can aid in differentiating the two.

Any client who displays an abnormality in mood, behavior, or cognition should be appropriately referred for further evaluation.

MEDICAL CONDITIONS
Diagnoses
Management
Knowledge
Compliance
Review client's diagnoses and determine client's awareness and understanding of medical conditions, ability to meet self-care requirements imposed by conditions, reactions to living with conditions, and compliance. Identify needs for education, counseling, assistive devices, financial aid, and other resources.

---

client's level of comfort during the assessment. Rapport must be established first. Many elderly have had little experience being interviewed and are less open than today's younger generation in discussing body functions, social problems, and feelings. They need to understand why this information is being requested, how it will benefit their care, and that it will be respected and held in confidence. Clients should be advised that they can freely ask questions or seek clarification of terms they do not understand. Staff members should remember that more time may be needed to assess older persons to allow for slower responses and review of the longer life histories they possess. Memory may be poor and special hints to trigger recall are sometimes needed. For example, instead of asking if an elderly person has any allergies, it may be more fruitful to ask if he/she has ever become sick or developed a rash from eggs, tomatoes, any other food, drugs, lotions, or materials. The ability to recall information can be further impaired by the stress of being interviewed or the admission process. Sensitivity is needed if clients have problems remembering information they should readily know; rather than dwelling on the unanswered question, return to it later. Avoid jargon that clients may not understand and compensate for sensory deficits that could interfere with effective communication.

Environmental factors can affect the assessment positively and negatively:

- *Distractors:* The area used to perform the assessment should afford privacy and not be in the midst of noise and traffic that could act as distractors. The assessment should not be conducted within hearing of others. If the client is in a semiprivate room, he/she should be taken to a private area for the assessment; if this is not possible, the curtain should be pulled between the beds and the nurse should sit on the side of the bed that is farthest away from the roommate's bed so that the client is less aware of the presence of the roommate.

- *Temperature:* The sensitivity of older persons to lower environmental temperatures could reduce their ability to be attentive and comfortable if the room is too cool. (This includes not only cool rooms on winter days but also cool inside temperatures created by air conditioners placed on low settings.) A room temperature of 75°F (24°C) is usually adequate; however, since individual differences and preferences exist, ask the client about the appropriateness of the temperature.

- *Glare:* Cataracts, a common finding in most older clients, cause bothersome glare from sources such as fluorescent lighting and direct sunlight through windows; controlling sources of glare and positioning the client so that he/she is not directly facing glare can facilitate comfort.

- *Bathroom facilities:* The frequent need of older adults to void necessitates that the assessment be conducted in an area in which a bathroom is easily accessible; the client should be informed of the location and offered the opportunity to toilet as needed.

- *Seating, positioning:* Seating should be arranged to allow approximately 4 feet between the client and the nurse; this provides an adequate social distance while being close enough to allow good visibility. The seating should provide comfort and support. The nurse should consider comfort measures and the need for position changes if the client is to lie on a hard examining table or chair for an extended period of time.

Most of the senses are used in performing an assessment:

- *Sight:* General appearance, grooming and hygienic practices, appropriateness and style of clothing, posture, deformities, body language, and limitations in function can be observed on initial visualization of the client.
- *Hearing:* Not only are responses and verbalized history heard but also the nurse's ears can detect problems such as the clicking of poorly fitting dentures, wheezes, coughs, and unusual voice quality.
- *Smell:* Odors may reflect poor hygienic practices, incontinence, discharge, infectious processes, alcohol use, acidosis, or liver disease. The decreased olfaction of many older persons can cause them to be unaware of such odors on themselves.
- *Touch:* By touch the nurse can determine skin temperature, turgor, painful sites, and the client's reaction to physical contact from others. Holding a hand, stroking a cheek, placing an arm around the shoulder, and using touch in other ways can communicate caring and interest by the nurse and facilitate the client's comfort with the assessment process.

The physical examination skills of inspection, auscultation, palpation, and percussion are used in the assessment. Nurses unfamiliar with physical assessment skills are advised to refer to texts on this topic for more depth and direction.

NURSING DIAGNOSIS AND PLANNING

The wealth of history and problems older people possess demands that the data collected be organized and prioritized so that appropriate care can be planned. Data should be analyzed for *existing* and *potential* problems. From these problems nursing diagnoses can be formulated.

A nursing diagnosis is a statement of a problem that nurses have the knowledge, skills, and legal authority to assess and manage. In that respect it differs from a medical diagnosis. Nurses are not prepared or legally able to derive a medical diagnosis, such as arthritis, but they can competently and legally manage the consequences of that medical condition, such as *pain* and *impaired physical mobility*. The problem, sign, or symptom is described in a standardized manner using the terminology listed in the NANDA-Approved Nursing Diagnostic Categories (Box 3-2); this is referred to as the diagnostic title. Using a nursing diagnosis allows the nurse to define the problem in a manner that can be diagnosed and treated within the realm of nursing.

A nursing diagnosis is a two-part statement:

Problem, sign, or symptom + Causative or contributing factor(s)

These components are linked by the phrase *related to*. The diagnostic title is the standardized, accepted stem of the diagnostic statement; the contributing or causative factor or factors can be numerous and rely on the nurse's assessment findings from the individual client; for example:

- Activity intolerance related to stiff joints and pain
- Activity intolerance related to depressed state
- Activity intolerance related to dizziness secondary to medication

These examples demonstrate that the contributing or causative factor is important to distinguish because interventions will differ significantly with each reason behind the diagnosis. Once the diagnostic statement is made, care can be planned accordingly. In fact, the construction of a good nursing diagnosis facilitates care planning in defining the specific problem that must be addressed. Table 3-2 gives examples of potential risks for the older client and possible related nursing diagnoses.

The care plan describes the goals and nursing interventions that address the identified nursing diagnoses. Ideally, a goal and specific nursing interventions should be described for each nursing diagnosis. A goal describes the outcome that is desired from nursing interventions. A well-written goal has the following characteristics:

BOX 3-2   NANDA-Approved Nursing Diagnostic Categories

PATTERN 1: EXCHANGING
Airway clearance, ineffective
Aspiration, high risk for
Body temperature, altered: high risk for
Bowel incontinence
Breathing pattern, ineffective
Cardiac output, altered: decreased
Constipation
Constipation, colonic
Constipation, perceived
Diarrhea
Disuse syndrome, high risk for
Dysreflexia
Fluid volume, altered: excess
Fluid volume deficit: actual
Fluid volume deficit: high risk for
Gas exchange, impaired
Hyperthermia
Hypothermia
Incontinence, functional/reflex/stress/total/urge
Infection, high risk for
Injury, high risk for
Nutrition, altered: less/more than body requirements
Oral mucous membrane, altered
Poisoning, high risk for
Skin integrity, impaired: actual
Skin integrity, impaired: high risk for
Suffocation, high risk for
Thermoregulation, ineffective
Tissue integrity, impaired
Tissue perfusion, altered
Trauma, high risk for
Urinary elimination, altered
Urinary retention

PATTERN 2: COMMUNICATING
Verbal communication, impaired

PATTERN 3: RELATING
Family processes, altered
Parental role conflict

Continued.

BOX 3-2   NANDA-Approved Nursing Diagnostic Categories—cont'd

Parenting, altered: actual
Parenting, altered: high risk for
Role performance, altered
Sexual dysfunction
Sexuality patterns, altered
Social interaction, impaired
Social isolation

PATTERN 4: VALUING
Spiritual distress

PATTERN 5: CHOOSING
Adjustment, impaired
Coping, defensive
Coping, ineffective family: compromised/disabling
Coping, ineffective individual
Decisional conflict (specify)
Denial, ineffective
Health-seeking behaviors (specify)
Noncompliance (specify)

PATTERN 6: MOVING
Activity intolerance, actual
Activity intolerance, high risk for
Breastfeeding, ineffective
Diversionary activity deficit
Fatigue
Growth and development, altered
Health maintenance, altered
Home maintenance management, impaired
Mobility, impaired physical
Self-care deficit (specify)
Sleep pattern disturbance
Swallowing, impaired

PATTERN 7: PERCEIVING
Hopelessness
Neglect, unilateral
Powerlessness
Self-concept, disturbance in body image/personal identity, self-esteem
Self-esteem, chronic low/situational low
Sensory-perceptual alteration (specify)

BOX 3-2   NANDA-Approved Nursing Diagnostic Categories—cont'd

PATTERN 8: KNOWING
Knowledge deficit (specify)
Thought processes, altered

PATTERN 9: FEELING
Anxiety
Fear
Grieving, anticipatory/dysfunctional
Pain
Pain, chronic
Posttraumatic response
Rape trauma syndrome
Violence, high risk for: self-directed or directed at others

- *Client focused:* The desired outcome for the client to achieve is described rather than that which staff will achieve; that is, "the client consumes at least 75% of each meal," not "staff members feed at least 75% of each meal to client."
- *Measurable:* The outcome described should be specific enough that any staff member can evaluate if it has been achieved; for example, stating that "the client increases weight" can be judged by one nurse to have been achieved if the client gains 2 pounds, whereas another nurse may believe that a 10-pound weight gain is necessary to achieve the goal; by specifically stating the weight gain desired, "client gains at least 5 pounds," there is no question as to the client's success in meeting the goal.
- *Designated time period:* The time frame in which the goal is to be achieved should be stated so that the client's success in meeting the goal can be determined; for example, rather than just saying that "the client gains at least 5 pounds," it is better to state "client gains at least 5 pounds within 1 month."
- *Realistic:* A goal must be achievable or it is worthless; it is far better to have a less than scholarly written goal that is realistic than to lift a great-sounding goal from a text or software program that cannot be achieved.

TABLE 3-2   Nursing Diagnoses for the Older Patient

Potential risks resulting from age-related changes	Related nursing diagnoses
Memory deficits	Alteration in health maintenance
	Noncompliance
	High risk for injury
	Impaired home maintenance management
	Knowledge deficit
	Anxiety
	Disturbance in self-concept
	Impaired social interactions
Slower learning of new information	Altered health maintenance
	Noncompliance
	Knowledge deficit
	Anxiety
Being stereotyped	Anxiety
	Powerlessness
	Disturbance in self-concept
	Alteration in family process
	Impaired social interactions
Dehydration	Fluid volume deficit
	Impaired skin integrity
	Altered oral mucous membrane
	Constipation
	Altered urinary elimination
Hypothermia	Potential alteration in body temperature
	Ineffective thermal regulation
Infection	Altered health maintenance
	Altered nutrition: less than body requirements
	Impaired skin integrity
	Activity intolerance
	Sleep pattern disturbance
	Pain
	Social isolation
Poor circulation	High risk for infection
	Impaired skin integrity
	Activity intolerance
	Altered tissue perfusion
Reduced gas exchange	High risk for infection
	Activity intolerance
	Ineffective airway clearance
	Ineffective breathing patterns
	Impaired gas exchange
	Altered thought processes

TABLE 3-2   Nursing Diagnoses for the Older Patient—cont'd

Potential risks resulting from age-related changes	Related nursing diagnoses
Aspiration	High risk for infection
	Ineffective airway clearance
	Impaired gas exchange
	Pain
	Anxiety
	Fear
Anorexia	Fluid volume deficit
	High risk for infection
	Altered nutrition: less than body requirements
	Constipation
	Altered thought processes
Indigestion	Altered nutrition: less than body requirements
	Pain
Constipation	Altered nutrition: less than body requirements
	Constipation
	Pain
Malabsorption of nutrients	High risk for infection
	Altered nutrition: less than body requirements
	Activity intolerance
	Impaired physical mobility
Delayed absorption, metabolism, and excretion of drugs	High risk for injury
	Self-care deficit
	Knowledge deficit
	Altered thought processes
Urinary frequency and urgency	High risk for injury
	Fluid volume deficit
	Impaired skin integrity
	Altered urinary elimination
	Sleep pattern disturbance
	Anxiety
	Disturbance in self-concept
	Social isolation
	Reflex incontinence
Stress incontinence	Functional incontinence
	High risk for injury
	Impaired skin integrity
	Altered urinary elimination
	Diversional activity deficit
	Anxiety

Continued.

TABLE 3-2   Nursing Diagnoses for the Older Patient— cont'd

Potential risks resulting from age-related changes	Related nursing diagnoses
	Disturbance in self-concept
	Social isolation
Prostatic hypertrophy	High risk for infection
	Altered urinary elimination
	Sleep pattern disturbance
	Anxiety
	Disturbance in self-concept
	Altered sexuality patterns
Senile vaginitis	Impaired skin integrity
	Pain
	Altered sexuality patterns
Dyspareunia	Pain
	Anxiety
	Disturbance in self-concept
	Sexual dysfunction
Fractures	Altered health maintenance
	High risk for injury
	Impaired skin integrity
	Activity intolerance
	Diversional activity deficit
	Impaired home maintenance management
	Impaired physical mobility
	Self-care deficit
	Alteration in comfort: pain
	Anxiety
	Powerlessness
	Disturbance in self-concept
	Sexual dysfunction
Immobility; range of motion	Altered health maintenance
	High risk for injury
	High risk for infection
	Impaired skin integrity
	Constipation
	Activity intolerance
	Ineffective breathing patterns
	Diversional activity deficit
	Impaired home maintenance management
	Impaired physical mobility
	Self-care deficit

TABLE 3-2   Nursing Diagnoses for the Older Patient—cont'd

Potential risks resulting from age-related changes	Related nursing diagnoses
	Powerlessness
	Disturbance in self-concept
	Social isolation
Muscle tremors and cramps	Activity intolerance
	Impaired physical mobility
	Sleep pattern disturbance
	Pain
Skin breakdown	High risk for infection
	Impaired skin integrity
	Pain
	Disturbance in self-concept

Nursing interventions should be developed that describe as specifically as possible those actions nursing staff will take to assist the client in meeting goals. A review of the plan with other disciplines and the development of multidisciplinary goals and actions promote efficient, comprehensive care. The client and significant others should participate in the development of the care plan and understand the goals and interventions that are planned.

The care plan is a working tool for all staff members to use in providing care to the client. As the client's condition changes, the care plan should be altered accordingly. Also, the care plan should be readily accessible to all nursing staff, and additions and changes to the plan communicated to all care givers.

IMPLEMENTATION

Perhaps the strongest area of nursing practice has been implementation because traditionally nurses have been taught the procedures involved in providing care. However, this phase of the nursing process can only be as strong as the phases preceding it. Nursing actions should support the care plan established.

Working with older adults requires some adjustments to nursing practice, such as the following:
- Activities take longer than they would for younger clients; therefore more time is needed for similar tasks.

- Age-related changes can alter the norms used to assess health status and the older client's responses to care, requiring that staff members be knowledgeable of and compensate for these differences.
- Advanced age heightens the risk of injury, infection, and other complications, necessitating active prevention of these adverse consequences.
- Older adults are more likely to have physical and psychosocial problems that affect each other and the outcome of care, demanding the use of a wide range of health, medical, social, and economic resources.
- Elderly individuals are likely to require the support and assistance of family care givers, thereby expanding nursing interventions to the total family unit.

EVALUATION

Evaluation is an ongoing and "fine tuning" phase in which necessary adjustments to care are detected and made. Evaluation is done informally during care activities and formally, at designated intervals, to determine if desired outcomes have been achieved (e.g., every 30 or 90 days). Nurses must consider not only if the desired results were achieved but also if they were achieved most effectively and efficiently for the client, the family, and all care givers. For example, hourly reality orientation of a demented client may not be totally beneficial if those hourly encounters cause agitation; likewise, assisting a terminally ill man to die in his home may need to be reevaluated if this plan is causing the care giver–wife considerable physical and emotional stress. All variables must be considered.

• • •

Underlying all phases of the nursing process is the philosophy that the client is to be assisted in achieving the highest maximum level of function possible. Approaches must be included that reduce or eliminate limitations to independent function and increase the capacity of the client for self-care.

Throughout all phases of care activities the rights of the client must be remembered and respected. Clients have the right to be informed of their care needs and activities, to refuse care, and to participate in care planning and delivery activities to the fullest degree possible.

RECOMMENDED READINGS

Burggraf V, Mickey S: *Nursing and the elderly: a care plan approach,* Philadelphia, 1989, Lippincott.

Duffy ME, MacDonald E: Determinants of functional health of older persons, *Gerontologist* 30:503, 1990.

Eliopoulos C, editor: *Health assessment of the older adult,* ed 2, Redwood City, CA, 1990, Addison-Wesley.

Eliopoulos C: *Resident assessment handbook: a guide for using the MDS,* Glen Arm, MD, 1991, Health Education Network.

Fields SD: History-taking in the elderly: obtaining useful information, *Geriatrics,* 46(8):36, 1991.

Maas M, Buckwalter K, Hardy M: *Nursing diagnosis and new interventions for the elderly,* Redwood City, CA, 1991, Addison-Wesley.

Naylor MD: Comprehensive discharge planning for hospitalized elderly: a pilot study, *Nurs Res* 39:156, 1990.

Teng EL, Chui HC: The modified mini-mental state examination, *J Clin Psychiatry* 48(8):314, 1987.

Walker SN: Wellness and aging. In Baines EM, editor: *Perspectives on gerontological nursing,* Newbury Park, CA, 1991, SAGE.

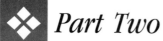 *Part Two*

Functional
Health Patterns

4

❖ Health Perception and Health Management

Older adults face unique challenges to maintaining health. Common aging changes can alter many body functions and increase the risk of health problems. These changes can alter norms and complicate the prompt identification of health problems. The stresses associated with retirement, widowhood, reduced income, and feeling more vulnerable and out of place in a youth-oriented society can weaken reserves and reduce motivation to engage in sound health practices. The misbelief that health deviations are an expected consequence of growing old may cause some older persons to accept and live with conditions that could be corrected or improved.

The high prevalence of chronic conditions presents another challenge to health maintenance in old age. It is the rare older adult who is free from chronic illness; more typically, the norm is for the older person to have several chronic illnesses. When one lives with a chronic illness, health assumes a different meaning. Rather than freedom from disease or a state of physical, emotional, or social well-being, a positive health state to a chronically ill person may be judged as being able to move fingers sufficiently to feed oneself, having ample energy to walk three blocks instead of just one, or being less lightheaded from medication. Management of chronic illness can be a large hurdle to overcome. New knowledge and skills may need to be gained. Daily life may be modified because of limitations and care requirements imposed by illness. The expense of medications and visits to the health care provider can create a financial burden. Leisure activities and social contacts may shrink. Health, a condition frequently taken for granted during earlier years, gradually develops into a significant concern and potentially a major obstacle to a satisfying life-style.

❖ **Generic Care Plan:**
ALTERED HEALTH MAINTENANCE
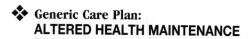

GENERAL INFORMATION

Altered health maintenance is the inability to identify or engage in practices and/or seek resources to maintain health. The individual is at risk because of inadequate preventive measures or an unhealthy life-style.

CAUSATIVE/CONTRIBUTING FACTORS

Alterations in communication skills
Perceptual or cognitive impairment
Lack of finances
Lack of motor skills
Unachieved developmental tasks
Changing support systems
Loss of independence
Lack of knowledge
Poor learning skills
Forced change (e.g., relocation)
Inadequate health practices
Religious, cultural, and health beliefs
Crisis situation
Substance abuse

CLINICAL MANIFESTATIONS

History of lack of health-seeking behavior
Lack of equipment, finances, personal support
Inability to take responsibility for meeting health needs
Lack of knowledge regarding health practices
Lack of access to health care services

NURSING PROCESS

Assessment Considerations
- General health status
- Presence of progressive illness or a long-term health problem
- Recent change in life-style
- Degree of independence or dependence
- Self-care ability
- Performance of activities of daily living (ADL)
- Cognition; emotional state
- Motor skills
- Knowledge and skills related to health maintenance
- Communication skills
- Income and expenses
- Support systems

Goals
- Client describes factor or factors responsible for altered health maintenance.
- Client identifies at least one way to improve health maintenance.
- Client engages in practices that meet at least minimum needs of respiration, nutrition, elimination, activity, rest, hygiene, and safety and is free from deficits related to each of these needs.

Nursing Interventions
- Provide health counseling and education to improve or correct identified problems, such as an unsafe home, unresolved grieving, nutritional deficits, poor vision or hearing, and altered bowel and bladder habits.
- Assist client in fulfilling self-care needs as necessary and appropriate.
- Teach and encourage good oral hygiene practices and dental checkups every 6 to 12 months.
- Identify self-care deficits, and, with client, develop a care plan to correct or improve deficits.
- Instruct client in self-examination techniques, such as breast and testicle examinations, and in signs to observe that could indicate illness.

- Recommend health screening at appropriate intervals:

Recommended Routine Health Screening

Annually: Breast examination, mammogram, stool for occult blood, digital rectal examination, tonometry, blood pressure
Every 2 years: General vision, hearing
Every 3 years: Pap smear, pelvic examination

- Recommend vaccinations at appropriate intervals:

Recommended Vaccination Schedule

Influenza: Annually
Pneumonia: Once in lifetime
Tetanus: Every 10 years

- Teach stress management skills.
- Refer to resources as necessary (e.g., substance abuse therapy, rehabilitation services, social services, home care).

Evaluation
- Client demonstrates positive state of health.
- Client demonstrates positive health practices (e.g., ingestion of appropriate diet, proper hygiene).
- Client appropriately uses resources to fulfill health needs.

Possible Related Nursing Diagnoses
Activity intolerance
Altered family processes
Altered role performance
Altered thought processes
Impaired home maintenance management
Impaired verbal communication
Ineffective individual coping
Infection, high risk for
Knowledge deficit
Noncompliance
Self-care deficit

❖ Generic Care Plan:
NONCOMPLIANCE

GENERAL INFORMATION

Noncompliance is personal behavior that deviates from health-related advice given by health care professionals.

CAUSATIVE/CONTRIBUTING FACTORS

Impaired physical function
Altered cognition, mood
Lack of or insufficient support systems
Insufficient finances
Insufficient knowledge
Poor motivation
Complex or overwhelming care demands

CLINICAL MANIFESTATIONS

Lack of improvement or worsening of health status
Missed appointments with health care provider
Failure to adhere to prescribed diet, drug regimens
Not obtaining prescriptions or supplies
Continuance of poor health practices (e.g., smoking, drinking)

NURSING PROCESS

Assessment Considerations
- General health and functional status
- Self-care ability
- Cognition, emotional state
- Support system
- Knowledge of health practices
- Motivation
- Income and expenses
- Responsibilities
- Available resources

Goals
- Client demonstrates improvement of health status.
- Client takes medications, performs treatments, adheres to diet, and so on as prescribed.
- Client keeps appointments with health care provider.

Nursing Interventions
- Assist client in finding means to reduce causative/contributing factor in ways such as the following:
    Obtaining financial aid
    Arranging for transportation
    Modifying environment
    Obtaining assistive devices, eyeglasses, hearing aid, walker
    Teaching stress reduction and management techniques
- Provide counseling and education regarding care requirements and reinforce importance of adhering to care plan.
- Encourage client to express feelings and concerns.

Evaluation
- Client demonstrates improvement in health status.
- Client adheres to care plan.
- Client uses resources, as needed, to comply with care requirements.

Possible Related Nursing Diagnoses
Altered family processes
Altered health maintenance
Altered thought processes
Anxiety
Fear
Hopelessness
Impaired physical mobility
Impaired verbal communication
Ineffective individual coping
Knowledge deficit
Powerlessness
Self-care deficit
Sensory-perceptual alteration
Social isolation

❖ Generic Care Plan:
HIGH RISK FOR INJURY

GENERAL INFORMATION

High risk for injury is a state in which an individual is at risk for accidental injury or trauma because of perceptual or physiologic deficit, lack of awareness, or advanced age.

CAUSATIVE/CONTRIBUTING FACTORS

Age-related changes (vision, coordination, reaction time)
Altered mobility
Altered cognition
Impaired sensory function
Pain
Fatigue, weakness
Poor coordination
Emotional disturbances
Poor knowledge of or adherence to safe practices
Unfamiliar environment (e.g., newly admitted to health care facility)
Environmental hazards (e.g., unsafe walkways, faulty electric wires, throw rugs, slippery floor, smoking in bed, clutter, gas leaks, malfunctioning appliances)
Inattentive, unskilled, or abusive care giver
Improper use of cane, walker, wheelchair, or other aids
Inappropriate use of hot water bottles, heating pads, enemas, soaks
Failure to use side rails on bed
Poor transfer and lifting techniques
Delayed or inappropriate response to accident or complication (e.g., not seeking medical examination after a fall, not reporting adverse drug reaction)

CLINICAL MANIFESTATIONS

History of accidents
Motor or sensory deficits
Presence of environmental hazards

Poor knowledge of safety practices
Evidence of physical injury (e.g., bruise, burn, limp)
Evidence of psychologic injury (e.g., withdrawal, behavioral change)

NURSING PROCESS

Assessment Considerations
- General health status
- Mobility
- Cognition
- Sensory function
- Self-care ability
- Knowledge of safety practices
- Environment
- Care-giver competency, relationship
- Use of wheelchair, cane, hearing aid, eyeglasses, and other assistive aids

Goals
- Client is free from injury.
- Client is able to identify safety risks and take actions to reduce or eliminate them.

Nursing Interventions
- Increase client's ability to protect self by the following:
    Obtaining eyeglasses, hearing aids, canes, walkers
    Improving general health status
    Educating and counseling
    Orienting to new surroundings
    Supporting treatment plan to improve underlying problem
- Provide supervision for client with altered cognition.
- Refer to ophthalmologist, audiologist, physical therapist, and other resources as needed.
- Assist with relocation if current living arrangements are hazardous.
- Instruct in measures to promote safety, such as transfer and ambulation techniques and safe medication use.
- Remove hazards from the environment:
    Arrange for correction of electrical, plumbing, heating, and appliance problems.

Arrange for homemaker through social service or private agency.

Assist in obtaining grab bars in tubs, handrails, and bed rails.

Ensure hot water heater temperature is not excessive.

- Teach client tips on preventing accidents, methods to fall safely, and emergency measures when accidents do occur.
- Provide for education to care giver as needed.

Evaluation

- Client identifies safety risks and takes appropriate action to protect self against injury.
- Client is free from injury.

Possible Related Nursing Diagnoses

Activity intolerance

Altered health maintenance

Altered thought processes

Fatigue

Impaired home maintenance management

Impaired physical mobility

Impaired verbal communication

Incontinence

Knowledge deficit

Self-care deficit

Sensory-perceptual alteration

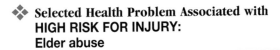

❖ Selected Health Problem Associated with HIGH RISK FOR INJURY: Elder abuse

GENERAL INFORMATION

Elder abuse consists of physical, emotional, sexual, or financial harm against an older individual or the threat of committing such actions. Many cases of abuse result from care-giver stress that weakens the care-giver's ability to cope. Although all states have laws related to elder abuse, most elderly are reluctant to report this problem because of embarassment or fear of repercussions.

CAUSATIVE/CONTRIBUTING FACTORS

Care-giver stress
Poor care giver–client relationship
Demanding, demented, hostile client
History of use of violence

CLINICAL MANIFESTATIONS

Unexplained bruise, burn, or injury
Report of mistreatment, injury, theft, or rape
Deprivation of food, care, medications, or services
Client's reluctance or fear to speak to professionals or neighbors
Signs of stress
Decline in physical or mental status

ADDITIONAL NURSING INTERVENTIONS TO INCORPORATE INTO GENERIC CARE PLAN

- Explore cause of unexplained injuries or subtle indications of mistreatment to help identify potential abuse.
- Assess relationship between client and persons with close relationship to client.
- Assist client and care giver in finding resources to ease care-giving burden.
- Explain legal rights and options available to abused client.
- Report all suspected or actual abuse to appropriate official agency; do not worry about repercussions; there is usually immunity for parties reporting abuse.

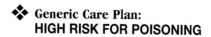 Generic Care Plan:
HIGH RISK FOR POISONING

GENERAL INFORMATION

High risk for poisoning exists when the client has an accentuated risk of accidental exposure to or ingestion of drugs or dangerous products in doses sufficient to cause harm.

CAUSATIVE/CONTRIBUTING FACTORS

Altered sensory function (e.g., poor vision, decreased olfaction)
Altered cognition
Improper use of medications (e.g., incorrect medication, dosage, route, or procedure)
Lack of knowledge or misinformation

CLINICAL MANIFESTATIONS

Inadequate knowledge of medications and their proper use
Polypharmacy
Evidence of illicit drugs or their use
Evidence of exposure to hazardous chemicals
Inappropriate use of substances (e.g., ingesting product intended for topical use)
Poor safety practices

NURSING PROCESS

Assessment Considerations

- Cognition
- Sensory function
- Self-care ability
- Types of prescription and nonprescription drugs used
- Knowledge of medications, proper use of chemicals
- Self-treatment measures used
- Environment, including storage of hazardous products
- Support systems

Goals

- Client is free from accidental poisoning.
- Client uses drugs appropriately.

Nursing Interventions

- Ensure medications are prescribed only when necessary and in appropriate dosages (recognizing need for age-adjusted levels); use nonpharmacologic alternatives when possible.
- Educate clients and care givers in safe use of medications (purpose, dosage, route, interactions, side effects); advise against self-prescription and altering dosages.

- For cognitively impaired clients, safeguard environment to prevent injury (e.g., lock up medications and noningestible substances, supervise activities, and observe closely).
- Administer medications appropriately; be aware of potential interactions.
- Ensure hazardous substances are clearly labelled.
- Caution client to store drugs or potentially poisonous substances in their original containers.
- Clarify misconceptions regarding inappropriate use of substances and home remedies.

Evaluation
- Client is free from adverse effects of medications.
- Client uses drugs as directed.
- Client stores medications and poisonous substances properly.

Possible Related Nursing Diagnoses
Altered health maintenance
Altered thought processes
Impaired home maintenance management
Knowledge deficit
Noncompliance
Self-care deficit
Sensory-perceptual alteration

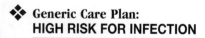

❖ **Generic Care Plan:**
   HIGH RISK FOR INFECTION

GENERAL INFORMATION

Older adults are at particularly high risk for developing infections. With advanced age, there is an altered antigen-antibody response, arising from atrophy of the thymus gland and reticuloendothelial system, defects in proliferation of lymphocytes, and decreased immunoglobulin production. Older adults have a high prevalence of chronic diseases (e.g., diabetes, chronic obstructive pulmonary disease [COPD]), which contribute to the high risk for infection. Age-related changes contribute to conditions that ease the path for infections to develop; such changes include the following:

- Decreased respiratory activity and ability to remove secretions from the lungs; reduced cough efficiency
- Weaker bladder muscles, leading to urinary retention and infection
- Prostatic hypertrophy and infection
- Increased alkalinity of vaginal secretions
- Fragility of skin and mucous membranes

Also older adults spend more time in hospitals and nursing homes than other age groups, predisposing them to the risk for nosocomial infections.

Infections not only develop easily in older adults but also are more difficult to identify early because of altered symptoms. For instance, the lower normal body temperature of many elderly persons can cause fever to exist at lower temperatures than what would be expected in the general population. Likewise, altered cognition, rather than chest pain and coughing, may be a primary sign of pneumonia.

CAUSATIVE/CONTRIBUTING FACTORS

Altered antigen-antibody reaction
Age-related changes
Disease (e.g., diabetes, cancer)
Immobility
Urinary catheter use
Malnutrition
Immunosuppressive or radiation therapy
Poor hygienic practices
Poor hand-washing and infection control practices of care
   givers

CLINICAL MANIFESTATIONS

Elevated temperature
Altered cognition
Aches and pain
Fatigue or malaise
Loss of appetite; weight loss
Urinary frequency, burning, or urgency
Discharge or itching
Cough or abnormal sputum characteristics
Foul odor

Lesions or ulcerated or reddened skin
Stiff, swollen joints

NURSING PROCESS

Assessment Considerations
- General health status
- Vital signs
- Cognition and behavior
- Appetite
- Energy level
- Presence of high-risk factors (e.g., immobility, frailty, urinary catheter, or disease)
- History of signs and symptoms of infection
- History of exposure to person with infection
- Knowledge of measures to prevent infection (e.g., proper toileting cleansing technique, hand washing, food storage, and housecleaning)

Goals
- Client is free from infection.
- Client verbalizes knowledge of and practices infection prevention measures.

Nursing Interventions
- Encourage good nutritional status by ensuring adequate intake of protein and vitamins.
- Promote fluid intake of at least 2000 ml daily, unless contraindicated, to lessen chance of dehydration and electrolyte imbalance.
- Monitor vital signs, mental status, intake and output, and general status.
- Adhere to proper hand-washing and hygienic practices and aseptic technique where applicable.
- Avoid use of urinary catheters unless absolutely necessary.
- Handle and store food properly.
- Maintain skin integrity and promote good skin care (see "Impaired skin integrity" in Chapter 5).
- Prevent client's exposure to persons with communicable diseases.
- Be alert to signs and symptoms that could indicate infection (e.g., subnormal body temperature, confusion, referred pain).

- Ensure client obtains pneumococcal vaccine once and influenza vaccine annually, unless contraindicated.
- Offer periodic tuberculosis screening for high-risk elderly who are institutionalized, exposed to large groups, or living in poor conditions (see discussion of tuberculosis on p. 155).
- Maintain a clean environment and handle wastes carefully.
- Instruct clients in good oral hygiene practices; assist as needed.
- Educate client about household cleaning; refer to homemaker's service if necessary.
- Educate client about proper food storage, cooking, and handling.
- Keep clients and their clothing and linens clean and dry.
- Offer massages or cold compresses for headaches.
- Administer antibiotics and analgesics as ordered; note precautions and interactions (Box 4-1; Table 8-1); monitor closely for adverse reactions.
- Obtain and communicate to physician results of laboratory specimens in a timely manner.
- Adhere to isolation procedures, if ordered.
- Note signs of new infections (e.g., diarrhea, moniliasis); superinfections can develop from long-term use of antibiotics.

Evaluation
- Client is free from signs of infection.
- Client practices measures to prevent or control infection.

Possible Related Nursing Diagnoses
Activity intolerance
Altered body temperature (high risk for)
Altered nutrition
Altered thought processes
Diarrhea
Fatigue
Fluid volume deficit
Impaired skin integrity
Incontinence
Ineffective breathing pattern
Knowledge deficit
Pain
Sleep pattern disturbance

BOX 4-1   Review of Selected Antibiotics

AMPICILLIN, CARBENICILLIN

Possible adverse effects

Rash, fever, chills, diarrhea, nausea, vomiting, irritations of mouth or tongue

Nursing implications

- Ask client about history of allergic reaction to penicillin; ensure drug is not given if allergy exists.
- Clients with altered renal or liver function may require reduced dosages.
- If antibiotic is administered orally, have client avoid food intake 2 hours before and 2 hours after administration.
- If antibiotic is administered intravenously, change site every 48 hours or as recommended by agency policy to avoid vein irritation.
- Instruct client who is self-administering ampicillin to follow these instructions:
    Avoid food intake 2 hours before and 2 hours after administration
    Continue taking drug for number of days prescribed even if symptoms subside
    Call physician if side effects develop
    Do not save unused drug
- Monitor serum potassium because high sodium content of drug can cause hypokalemia.
- Interactions: Effects are decreased by antacids, chloramphenicol, erythromycin, tetracycline.

CEFACLOR, CEPHALORIDINE

Possible adverse effects

Rash, headache, drowsiness, dizziness, nausea, vomiting, indigestion, diarrhea, abdominal cramping, irritation of mouth or tongue

Nursing implications

- Ask client about history of allergic reaction to any cephalosporin; ensure drug is not given if allergy exists. Also ask about allergic reaction to penicillin because persons with this allergy are at higher risk of allergic reaction to cephalosporins.
- Since cephalosporins are nephrotoxic, use with care in persons with impaired renal function.
- Observe for superinfections.
- Drug may be administered with meals.
- Review client's ability to purchase drug; cephalosporins are more expensive than other antibiotics.
- Interactions: effects are increased by probenecid.

DOXYCYCLINE

Possible adverse effects

Rash, anorexia, nausea, vomiting, diarrhea, irritation of mouth or tongue

BOX 4-1 Review of Selected Antibiotics—cont'd

Nursing implications
- Do not expose drug to light or heat.
- Administer with meals or milk.
- Drug can alter results of Clinitest and similar urine tests.
- There is a high risk of thrombophlebitis with intravenous administration.
- Interactions: Absorption is decreased when administered with aluminum, calcium- or magnesium-based laxatives, antacids, iron preparations, phenobarbital, or alcohol.

ERYTHROMYCIN
Possible adverse effects
Rash, hives, nausea, vomiting, diarrhea, liver damage with long-term use

Nursing implications
- Erythromycin estolate is contraindicated in persons with impaired liver function; can cause hepatotoxicity.
- Coated tablets can be taken with meals; otherwise patient should take medication 2 hours before or 2 hours after eating.
- Tablets should be followed by at least 8 ounces of water; do not administer with juices.
- Interactions: Penicillins will antagonize effects of erythromycin and vice versa; do not give penicillin within 2 hours of erythromycin; levels of theophylline, warfarin, methylprednisolone, and carbamazepine can be increased by erythromycin.

KANAMYCIN
Possible adverse effects
Headache, nausea, vomiting, tinnitus, vertigo, hearing loss (ototoxicity)

Nursing implications
- Use with extreme caution in elderly because of nephrotoxicity.
- Monitor renal function closely (e.g., intake and output, weight, blood urea nitrogen [BUN]).
- Encourage good fluid intake to help reduce concentration of kanamycin in kidney tissue.
- Obtain baseline audiometric reading and reevaluate periodically throughout therapy.
- Toxic effects are more likely when blood level exceeds 30 μg/ml.

NITROFURANTOIN
Possible adverse effects
Dyspnea, coughing, asthma attacks, other respiratory problems

Continued.

BOX 4-1   Review of Selected Antibiotics—cont'd

Nursing implications
- Use is contraindicated in persons with impaired renal function.
- Administer with food or milk.
- Urine may become dark or brown (not significant); note intake and output.
- Discontinue at first sign of respiratory reaction; report to physician.
- Drug can cause false glycosuria readings with Clinitest.
- May take 1 to 2 weeks of therapy for noticeable response; evaluate urine specimens for culture and sensitivity periodically during therapy.
- Store in a dark, nonmetallic container.
- Interactions: Effects are increased by probenecid; effects are decreased by phenobarbital.

SULFISOXAZOLE
Possible adverse effects
Rash, anorexia, abdominal pain, irritation of mouth, tinnitus, tingling of extremities, delirium, bone marrow depression, hepatitis, kidney damage, hemolytic anemia (particularly if administered with isoniazid)

Nursing implications
- Ask about history of allergic reaction to any sulfonamide (sulfa drug); use is contraindicated if allergy exists.
- Use with caution in persons with liver or kidney disease or history of bronchial asthma or allergies.
- Take with a full glass of water; encourage good fluid intake to prevent crystals from forming in urine.
- Monitor intake and output.
- Urine may become dark or brown (not significant).
- If vitamin C is prescribed, consult with physician; vitamin C administered during therapy will make urine more acidic, contributing to crystal formation.
- Interactions: Drug increases effects of alcohol, oral anticoagulants, oral antidiabetic agents, methotrexate, phenytoin; it decreases effects of penicillin; effects are increased by aspirin, oxyphenbutazone, probenecid, promethazine, sulfinpyrazone, and trimethoprim; effects are decreased by paraldehyde, para-aminosalicylic acid.

RECOMMENDED READINGS

Besdone RW: Hyperthermia and accidental hypothermia. In Abrams WB, Berkow R, editors: *The Merck manual of geriatrics,* Rahway, NJ, 1990, Merck Sharp and Dohme Research Laboratories.

Bush LM, Kaye D: Epidemiology and pathogenesis of infectious diseases. In Abrams WB, Berkow R, editors: *The Merck manual of geriatrics,* Rahway, NJ, 1990, Merck Sharp and Dohme Research Laboratories.

Demarest GB, Osler TM, Clevenger FW: Injuries in the elderly: evaluation and initial response, *Geriatrics* 45(8):36, 1990.

Gerhart TN: Fractures. In Abrams WB, Berkow R, editors: *The Merck manual of geriatrics,* Rahway, NJ, 1990, Merck Sharp and Dohme Research Laboratories.

Janz M: Clues to elder abuse, *Geriat Nurs* 11(5):220, 1990.

Ross KL: Meningitis as it presents in the elderly: diagnosis and care, *Geriatrics* 45(8):63, 1990.

Wolf RS, Pellemer KA: *Helping elderly victims: the reality of elder abuse,* New York, 1989, Columbia University Press.

5

Nutrition and Metabolism

Proper diet is especially important for older persons to promote optimal physical and mental function, strengthen the ability to prevent disease, and reduce secondary problems associated with existing chronic illnesses. Receiving adequate nutrients can become a major challenge to the elderly because of age-related changes in the digestive system (see Chapter 2) and lifelong dietary practices that may be less than ideal.

Nutritional requirements must be individually determined based on the client's height, weight, health status, and activity pattern. There are some general guidelines, however, that can be considered when planning nutritional needs. Caloric requirements are reduced in late life because of a lower metabolic rate, a less active state than existed in earlier years of life, and the proportionate increase in adipose tissue over lean tissue. The general recommendation is for older women to reduce their caloric intake to 1800 calories until 75 years of age and to 1600 calories thereafter; older men should limit calories to 2400 until 75 years of age and 2050 after that age. The calories consumed should represent high quality nutrients. Protein requirements remain fairly consistent throughout the life span: 56 g/day for males and 44 g/day for females. Intake of simple carbohydrates and saturated fats should be low.

The Metropolitan Life Insurance Company's weight scales, which in the past have provided guidelines for normal weight, have been replaced with new weight ranges from the Gerontology Research Center. The new weight ranges are age adjusted and show heavier normal weights with each decade through adulthood (see Table 3-1); these adjusted weight scales must be used when assessing nutritional status.

Vitamin and mineral requirements are consistent throughout the life span (Table 5-1) and usually can be met through the ingestion of a well-balanced diet of fruits, vegetables, and dairy products. Vitamin and mineral supplements may be indicated in cases of absorption problems, inadequate dietary intake, unusual stress, and healing. Megadoses have no proven benefit and may produce toxicities.

Fiber promotes good elimination and can be obtained through fruits, vegetables, and whole-grain breads and cereals. A daily intake of 30 to 60 g of fiber is recommended.

Total body fluids are reduced with age because of a reduction in intracellular fluids. The lower fluid reserve reduces the margin of safety that exists when fluid volume deficits exist.

TABLE 5-1 Recommended Daily Dietary Intake for Persons over Age 65

Nutrient	Recommended daily intake
Protein	56 g (men); 44 g (women)
Vitamin A	1000 g RE[1] (men); 800 g RE (women)
Vitamin B_1 (thiamine)	1.2 mg (men); 1 mg (women)
Vitamin B_2 (riboflavin)	1.4 mg (men); 1.2 mg (women)
Vitamin B_3 (niacin)	16 mg (men); 13 mg (women)
Vitamin B_6 (pyridoxine)	2.2 mg (men); 2 mg (women)
Vitamin B_{12} (cobalamin)	3 mg
Folacin	400 g
Vitamin C	60 mg
Vitamin D	5 g
Vitamin E	10 mg α-TE[2] (men); 8 mg α-TE (women)
Calcium	800 mg
Phosphorus	800 mg
Magnesium	350 mg (men); 300 mg (women)
Iodine	150 g
Iron	10 mg
Zinc	15 mg

Data from National Academy of Sciences: *Recommended daily dietary allowances,* Washington, DC, 1993, US Government Printing Office.
[1]Retinol equivalents.
[2]α = Tocopherol.

> ## BOX 5-1   Factors That Increase Risk of Nutritional Problems in the Elderly
>
> **PHYSIOLOGIC FACTORS**
> - Decreased secretion of enzymes; indigestion common
> - Decreased absorption of nutrients and minerals
> - Reduced mobility of stomach; slowing of peristalsis
> - Restricted intake of nutrients caused by problems with teeth and dentures (e.g., ill-fitting dentures, periodontal disease, missing teeth)
> - Decrease in production of saliva
> - Reduced sensitivity to sweet and salty flavors
> - Low activity level
> - Disease-related symptoms that can reduce appetite, energy, or ability to ingest food
> - Side effects of medications
>
> **PSYCHOSOCIAL FACTORS**
> - Limited finances that prohibit purchase of proper food
> - Lack of knowledge regarding nutritional needs, nutritional value of foods
> - Inability to shop, store foods, or cook (e.g., lack of transportation, no kitchen facilities, dementia)
> - Personal preferences that violate principles of good nutritional intake
> - Loneliness or eating alone
> - Mood disturbances (e.g., depression, anxiety)

Unless fluid restrictions are necessary, at least 2000 ml of fluid should be consumed daily.

Many factors can cause or contribute to altered nutrition in the elderly (Box 5-1). These factors must be reviewed during the assessment, and interventions planned to prevent or correct them should be implemented as necessary.

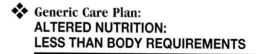

❖ Generic Care Plan:
ALTERED NUTRITION:
LESS THAN BODY REQUIREMENTS

GENERAL INFORMATION

Altered nutrition: less than body requirements exists when there is an insufficient intake of nutrients to meet body needs.

CAUSATIVE/CONTRIBUTING FACTORS

Knowledge deficit about nutritional needs

Age-related changes: decreased taste acuity, reduced sensitivity to thirst and hunger, decreased gastric secretions, reduced protein synthesis and turnover

Pain

Anorexia

Emotional stress

Depression

Dementia

Social isolation

Inability to procure or prepare food

Limited finances

Inability to ingest, digest, or absorb nutrients

Sore, inflamed buccal cavity

Treatments

CLINICAL MANIFESTATIONS

20% or more under ideal body weight

Weight loss of at least 5% in past month; at least 10% in past 6 months

Triceps skinfold or midarm circumference less than 60% of standard measurement

History of inadequate food intake

Muscle weakness and tenderness

Fatigue

Altered mental function; delirium

Evidence of reduced food intake

Aversion to eating

Diarrhea or hyperactive bowel sounds

Poor skin turgor or pallor

Capillary fragility

Altered laboratory findings: for example, low serum albumin, serum transferrin, hemoglobin, hematocrit, lymphocytes

NURSING PROCESS

Assessment Considerations

- Physical status

  Precise weight: using same scale, same amount of clothing, and same time of day each time weighed

  Vital signs

Triceps skinfold measurement, midarm circumference
Hair quantity and quality
Skin color, turgor, and integrity
Muscle tone and strength
Visual acuity, night vision, and moisture of eyes
Status of oral cavity, teeth/dentures
Taste and smell acuity
Swallowing
- Laboratory analysis of urine (specific gravity), blood (total iron binding capacity, transferrin saturation, protein, albumin, hemoglobin, hematocrit, electrolytes, vitamins, prothrombin time)
- Diet history
  Unusual or unhealthy eating habits (ask specific questions)
  Food likes, dislikes, restrictions, intolerances
  Use of alcohol and drugs (prescription and nonprescription)
- Food diary: record of times and type of intake
- Psychosocial factors (e.g., loneliness, lack of companionship)
- Cognition, mood, level of consciousness
- Ability to afford, shop for, prepare, and store food
- Existing health problems
- Medications or other treatments
- Recent losses and stresses

Goals
- Client gains ____ pounds within 1 month.
- Client has laboratory values that fall within the normal range.
- Client verbalizes good knowledge about nutrition.
- Client expresses satisfaction with diet.
- Client consumes at least 75% of each meal; consumes at least ____ calories/day.
- Client is free from signs of malnutrition.

Nursing Interventions
- Identify factors that cause or contribute to altered nutritional state.
- Consult with other health team members regarding measures to correct nutritional problems, for example, remove loose or diseased teeth, treat periodontal disease, replace dentures, prescribe appetite stimulants, initiate psychiatric consulation.
- Use assessment data to plan meals; avoid foods that cause intolerance or indigestion; offer preferred, culturally favored foods.
- Consult with physician and nutritionist regarding diet modifi-

cations: dietary supplements, high-protein or high-calorie diet, soft diet, use of appetite stimulants (e.g., small amount of wine).
- Assist client in incorporating special dietary needs/restrictions into usual pattern of eating; recognize that it is difficult for people to change lifelong eating patterns; offer compromises as needed to avoid complete rejection of special diet, and reward compliance with occasional treat as allowed within diet; encourage client to express feelings about dietary restrictions.
- Maintain record of food and fluid intake.
- Offer frequent, small meals.
- Encourage client to maximize nutrient content of each calorie ingested (e.g., a doughnut and a glass of milk may have the same amount of calories, but the milk will offer four times the amount of protein and minerals).
- Judge carbohydrate intake in relation to caloric needs; reduce intake of simple carbohydrates (e.g., sugar) and replace with complex carbohydrates (e.g., cereals, breads).
- Offer oral hygiene and opportunity for toileting before meals.
- Enhance food by using flavoring (lemon, herbs); promote optimal taste by instructing client to alternate mouthfuls of foods during meals (e.g., a mouthful of meat, then a mouthful of potatoes, then a mouthful of peas, then a mouthful of bread) because taste acuity for a given flavor will diminish as more of that same flavor is eaten.
- Promote a pleasant and relaxing atmosphere for eating; encourage and assist client in eating with others.
- Assist with feeding, as necessary; provide assistive devices to promote feeding independence.
- Allow adequate time for eating; feed slowly.
- Prevent early satiety by limiting fiber/bulk and fluid intake 1 hour before meals.
- Teach client importance of balanced diet and need for a consistent intake of nutrients to reach and maintain ideal weight.
- Caution client against factors that can interfere with absorption of nutrients (e.g., alcohol, tobacco).
- Arrange resources for client's use, such as Meals on Wheels or food stamps.
- Be alert to food-drug interactions (e.g., liver, spinach, turnip greens, cabbage, and broccoli can interfere with the effectiveness of oral anticoagulants; antacids can reduce the potency of oral antibiotics, digoxin, oral anticoagulants, and salicylates).
- Identify and act early on subtle signs of nutritional problems (Table 5-2).

TABLE 5-2   Signs of Nutritional Problems

Nutritional problem	Signs and symptoms
Vitamin A deficiency	Dry skin
	Persistent "goose bumps"
	Night blindness
Vitamin B_6 deficiency	Red, scaly skin (generalized)
	Burning feet
	Hypochromic anemia
	Depression
	Confusion
Vitamin C deficiency	Purpura
	Swollen, bleeding gums (if teeth present)
Vitamin D deficiency	Bone pain and tenderness
	Frequent or unexplained fractures
Vitamin K deficiency	Purpura
Iron deficiency	Pallor
	Weakness, fatigue
Magnesium deficiency	Vertigo
	Seizures
	Muscle weakness, tremors
	Depression, irritability
Niacin deficiency (pellagra)	Sore mouth
	Brownish pigmentation of skin exposed to light
	Dermatitis
	Diarrhea
	Confusion, depression
Phosphate deficiency	Fatigue, malaise
	Muscle weakness
	Bone pain
Potassium deficiency	Weakness
	Drowsiness
	Nausea, vomiting
Riboflavin deficiency	Red, scaly skin in folds around eyes and between nose and corners of mouth
	Fissures in corner of mouth
	Smooth, purple, and sore tongue
	Genital dermatitis
Zinc deficiency	Dermatitis, primarily in periphery of limbs
	Decreased taste sensation
	Delayed wound healing
Hyperglycemia	Recurrent boils, fungus infections
	Increased thirst, voiding, hunger
Hyperuricemia	Gout

Evaluation
- Client maintains weight between ⎯⎯ and ⎯⎯ pounds.
- Client gains ⎯⎯ pounds within 1 month.
- Client demonstrates necessary changes in eating patterns and food quality and quantity.
- Client consumes appropriate quantity and quality of nutrients.
- Client's laboratory values are within normal limits.

Possible Related Nursing Diagnoses
Activity intolerance
Actual or high risk for fluid volume deficit
Altered oral mucous membrane
Altered thought processes
Constipation
Diarrhea
Fatigue
High risk for infection
Impaired swallowing
Knowledge deficit: diet
Noncompliance: dietary
Self-care deficit: feeding
Sensory-perceptual alteration: gustatory, olfactory, visual

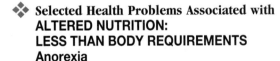

**❖❖ Selected Health Problems Associated with
ALTERED NUTRITION:
LESS THAN BODY REQUIREMENTS
Anorexia**

GENERAL INFORMATION

Anorexia refers to the loss of appetite and lack of interest in food.

CAUSATIVE/CONTRIBUTING FACTORS

Physical disease: for example, cancer, chronic obstructive pulmonary disease
Emotional illness: for example, depression, anxiety
Life crisis, grief
Social isolation
Inactivity
Medications

CLINICAL MANIFESTATIONS

Disinterest in food
Reduced food intake
Weight loss
Fatigue, weakness
Altered mental status

ADDITIONAL NURSING INTERVENTIONS
TO INCORPORATE INTO GENERIC PLAN

- Urge family and friends to prepare special meals that client is known to like.
- Provide good oral hygiene before and after meals.
- Provide meals in pleasant surroundings: promote socialization; remove bedpans, supplies, and litter; make client comfortable.
- Present food attractively: serve at correct temperatures; vary colors and textures; avoid styrofoam and plastic plates and utensils; have tablecloth and flowers on table; provide background music.
- Offer several smaller meals rather than a few large ones.
- Consult with nutritionist and physician regarding benefit of vitamin and mineral supplements, appetite stimulants.
- Consult with social service and psychiatric specialists regarding possible interventions.

Anemia

GENERAL INFORMATION

Anemia is a condition in which there is a reduced red blood cell count or subnormal hemoglobin or hematocrit level. This is a common finding in the older population, affecting about one third of the elderly, and is symptomatic of an underlying health problem.

CAUSATIVE/CONTRIBUTING FACTORS

Iron deficiency anemia. Most common form; may be caused by insufficient dietary intake of iron, impaired iron absorption, or excessive blood loss (e.g., from an ulcer, hemorrhoids, gastritis)

Pernicious anemia. Caused by impaired absorption of vitamin B_{12} or stomach cancer

Aplastic anemia. Serious, although less common, form of anemia that can be caused by radiation, chemicals (insecticides), or drugs (acetazolamide, antibiotics, anticonvulsants, antihistamines, chloramphenicol, chlorthiazide, nonsteroidal antiinflammatory agents, phenothiazines, sulfonamides)

CLINICAL MANIFESTATIONS

Pallor, often most noticeable in oral mucosa and conjunctiva

Fatigue

Dizziness

Headache

Poor skin turgor

Changes in mental status: confusion, depression, agitation

Increased cardiac output

Palpitations, worsening angina

Dyspnea, shortness of breath

Pernicious anemia

    Anorexia

    Smooth red tongue

    Gastrointestinal symptoms: indigestion, recurring diarrhea and constipation

    Weight loss

    Infection

Aplastic anemia

    Purpura

    Bleeding

ADDITIONAL NURSING INTERVENTIONS
TO INCORPORATE INTO GENERIC CARE PLAN

- Increase client's consumption of iron-rich foods (e.g., green leafy vegetables, meat, fish, poultry, dried fruits, enriched breads and cereals).
- Encourage vitamin C intake (ascorbic acid promotes iron absorption).
- Prepare client for side effects of iron supplements, such as indigestion, darker-colored stools, and constipation.
- Administer and observe for side effects of steroids and androgens if prescribed.

- Schedule rest periods between activities and treatments.
- Assist with blood transfusions, if ordered; monitor carefully for symptoms of transfusion reaction.

Cirrhosis

GENERAL INFORMATION

Cirrhosis is a progressive disease of the liver characterized by tissue scarring that ultimately results in severe liver failure and death. Cirrhosis increases in incidence in mid-life and is the ninth leading cause of death in the elderly.

CAUSATIVE/CONTRIBUTING FACTORS

Alcoholism (most often)
Hepatitis
Biliary obstruction

CLINICAL MANIFESTATIONS

Jaundice
Dark, rust-colored urine
Clay-colored stools
Portal hypertension
Bleeding tendencies
Edema and ascites
Drowsiness
Confusion
Reduced resistance to infection
Palpable spleen
Distended abdominal wall veins

ADDITIONAL NURSING INTERVENTIONS
TO INCORPORATE INTO GENERIC CARE PLAN

- Arrange for/assist with diagnostic tests: serum alkaline phosphatase, prothrombin time, hepatic scanning, liver biopsy.
- Administer folic acid and vitamins A, D, K, and B complex as ordered.

- Assist client in adhering to dietary modifications: high-protein, high-calorie, low-fat, sodium-restricted (if retaining fluid) diet; offer small meals frequently rather than large ones; encourage use of supplements.
- Maintain bed rest as needed and ordered.
- Consult with physician regarding need to adjust medication dosages (some drugs are metabolized in the liver).
- Monitor vital signs, edema, ascites, jaundice, mental status, level of consciousness (hepatic coma is a serious complication of this condition).
- Test every stool for occult blood.
- Offer regular skin care for cleansing, relief of pruritus.
- Offer or arrange for alcoholism treatment and counseling.

❖ **Generic Care Plan:**
ALTERED NUTRITION:
MORE THAN BODY REQUIREMENTS

GENERAL INFORMATION

Altered nutrition: more than body requirements is the state in which the intake of nutrients exceeds metabolic demand.

CAUSATIVE/CONTRIBUTING FACTORS

High-carbohydrate, high-calorie diet
Reduced activity
Depression, boredom
Metabolic abnormalities
Knowledge deficit regarding nutritional needs
Limited finances

CLINICAL MANIFESTATIONS

Weight at least 20% above ideal
Documented intake in excess of metabolic requirements
Evidence of unbalanced diet
Pattern of sedentary activity either enforced or by choice

NURSING PROCESS

Assessment Considerations
- Physical status
    - Precise weight: using same scale, same amount of clothing, and same time of day each time weighed
    - Vital signs
    - Triceps skinfold measurement, midarm circumference
    - Muscle tone and strength
    - Ability to chew, swallow, and digest diet
- Diet history
    - Unusual or unhealthy eating habits (ask specific questions)
    - Food likes, dislikes, restrictions, intolerances
    - Use of alcohol and drugs (prescription and nonprescription)
- Food diary: record of times and type of intake
- Psychosocial factors (e.g., use of food to deal with stress, anxiety, loneliness)
- Cognition, mood, level of consciousness
- Physical problems related to weight (e.g., decreased mobility, impaired skin integrity, fatigue, weakness)
- Client's feelings and perceptions about weight
- Ability to afford, shop for, prepare, and store food
- Existing health problems
- Medications and other treatments
- History of attempts at weight management

Goals
- Client reduces weight by ＿＿ pounds within 1 month.
- Client maintains weight between ＿＿ and ＿＿ pounds.
- Client expresses satisfaction with dietary restrictions and weight adjustment.
- Client verbalizes understanding of proper diet.

NURSING INTERVENTIONS
- Consult nutritionist to determine caloric needs and restrictions.
- Teach client and family about potential problems resulting in or from nutritional excess (e.g., disease process, medication side effects, impaired mobility).
- Reinforce dietary plans; provide counseling if client is ready to accept it in areas such as menu planning, identification of behaviors that lead to overeating, behavior modification, exercise.
- Facilitate compliance with prescribed diet by providing positive reinforcement.

- Help client develop a regimen to increase activity and decrease caloric consumption; provide a schedule that allows ample opportunity for physical activity; limit snacks.
- Provide emotional support for the family and client as they learn new behaviors (e.g., altered cooking methods, exercise, changed eating habits).
- Refer to psychologic or nutritional counseling, weight loss/support groups as necessary.

Evaluation
- Client loses ____ pounds per week/month.
- Client verbalizes knowledge of healthy eating habits.
- Client demonstrates compliance with dietary plan.
- Client establishes and adheres to a regularly scheduled activity program.

Possible Related Nursing Diagnoses
Activity intolerance
Disturbance in self-concept
Fatigue
Impaired physical mobility
Ineffective individual coping
Knowledge deficit related to diet
Noncompliance related to diet
Sleep pattern disturbance
Social isolation

 Selected Health Problems Associated with ALTERED NUTRITION: MORE THAN BODY REQUIREMENTS Diabetes mellitus

GENERAL INFORMATION

Diabetes mellitus is a chronic, hereditary disease characterized by a blood glucose level that exceeds normal most of the time. This problem results from a lack of insulin production (type 1) or production of insulin that is ineffective (a problem more common in the elderly) or insufficient to meet the body's demands (type 2). Problems in the metabolism of carbohydrates, protein, and fat result.

Usually, the presentation of symptoms raises suspicion that diabetes exists. Sometimes, diabetes is detected during the evaluation of other problems, such as orthostatic hypotension, stroke, gastric hypotony, neuropathy, impotence, Dupuytren's contracture, or glaucoma. Laboratory evaluation demonstrating elevated plasma glucose concentrations confirms the diagnosis. Normal increases in blood glucose levels with age require that age-related gradients be used to evaluate test results.

Diabetes first diagnosed at an older age may be controlled with diet alone or with oral hypoglycemic agents. Regular exercise is important and can reduce insulin requirements; immobility can cause a deterioration of glucose tolerance. Active prevention of complications (e.g., hypoglycemia, neuropathies, retinopathy, peripheral vascular disease, and infections) is an essential part of the care plan also.

CAUSATIVE/CONTRIBUTING FACTORS

Total or partial lack of insulin production
Increased demand for insulin (e.g., obesity)
Physiologic deterioration in glucose tolerance as a result of advanced age, immobility

CLINICAL MANIFESTATIONS

Fatigue, weakness
Drowsiness after meals
Weight loss
Polyuria or nocturia
Polyphagia
Polydipsia
Pruritus
Slow wound healing
Altered mental status
Easy development of infections
Blurred vision
Muscle cramps

ADDITIONAL NURSING INTERVENTIONS
TO INCORPORATE INTO GENERIC CARE PLAN

• If glucose tolerance testing is to be done, prepare client in advance.

Provide a high (at least 150-g) carbohydrate diet for several
    days beforehand.
Explain that blood will be drawn at regular intervals (before
    glucose administration and 1, 2, and 3 hours after.
Be alert to signs of unusual stress, illness, malnutrition, or
    inactivity before testing; report to physician.
Review medications being taken by the client; nicotinic acid,
    ethacrynic acid, estrogen, furosemide, and diuretics can
    decrease glucose tolerance and may be withheld before
    testing; high doses of salicylates may lower blood sugar
    levels and interfere with testing; consult with physician if
    these medications are being used.
Age-related gradients are used to interpret test findings.
Diagnosis of diabetes in older adults is made after client is
    found to have fasting blood glucose $\geq$ 140 mg, or 2-hour
    blood glucose level $\geq$ 200 mg.
Inform the client that several tests may be needed before the
    diagnosis is confirmed.
- Instruct the client in recognition of signs and symptoms of
  hyperglycemia and hypoglycemia (Box 5-2).
- Teach proper foot care by having client regularly exercise feet;
  inspect for abnormalities, discolorations, skin breaks, or change
  in temperature (Box 5-3).

BOX 5-2 Signs and Symptoms of Hyperglycemia and Hypoglycemia

HYPERGLYCEMIA
Dry mouth
Thirst
Sweet, fruity-smelling
    breath
Anorexia, nausea, vomiting
Excess voiding
Abdominal pain
As it progresses:
Disorientation
Labored breathing
Dry, flushed skin
Drowsiness
Coma
Death

HYPOGLYCEMIA
Confusion
Hunger
Tachycardia
Trembling
Weakness
Perspiration
Irritability
Tingling fingers, mouth
Headache
Appearance of being
    intoxicated
As it progresses:
Seizure
Stroke
Death

BOX 5-3 Foot Care Practices for the Diabetic Client

SPECIAL FOOT CARE

Is important for someone with diabetes because:

- Diabetes reduces the healthy blood flow to the feet so cuts take longer to heal and can easily lead to sores and infections.
- Diabetes can affect the nerves that signal when temperatures are too hot or too cold, thereby reducing the individual's ability to be aware of the threat of an injury.

DAILY FOOT CARE

Washing

- Wash the feet in warm water with a mild soap. Rinse well. Do not apply alcohol or soak the feet.
- Dry feet gently with a towel, especially between the toes.

Inspection

- After cleaning feet, examine them closely, including between the toes.
- If eyesight is not good, arrange for a family member or other care giver to inspect feet at least once each week.
- Look for dry skin, cracks, cuts, sores, change in color (red, blue, white), blisters, bruises.

Skin care

- After inspecting feet, apply lotion so skin does not become dry and cracked.
- Avoid the use of lotion between toes and around toenails.
- If feet sweat a lot, use a gentle foot powder after drying.

FOOTWEAR CONSIDERATIONS

- Wear shoes that fit well, are comfortable, have a low heel, and cover the foot. Cutout shoes, sandals, or pointed shoes increase risk of injury.
- Wear shoes or slippers around the house to avoid stubbing toes.
- Do not go barefoot.
- When shopping for shoes, make purchase at end of the day when feet are at their largest.
- Wear new shoes only ½ hour per day at first to break them in.
- Check inside of shoes for stones or torn linings before putting them on.
- Wear clean, white (to avoid sensitivity to dye) socks of wool or cotton; avoid nylon; change socks daily.
- Never wear socks that are tight and constrict the flow of blood; women should wear pantyhose or a garter belt rather than garters or knee-high hose.

CARING FOR TOENAILS

- Do not cut own nails if there are problems with vision, shaky hands, or trouble reaching the toes.

BOX 5-3   Foot Care Practices for the Diabetic Client—cont'd

- If nails are thick, cracked, or split, have a podiatrist care for them.
- Use nail clippers to cut nails straight across; do not cut into corners to make nails round.
- Do not cut a nail shorter than the edge of the toe.
- Gently file sharp edges and corners with an emery board.

PREVENTING ATHLETE'S FOOT
- This fungus infection grows in warm, moist places, so keep feet clean and dry.
- Use a foot powder to keep feet dry.
- Change socks if they become moist.
- Do not use any foot medication without consulting your physician.
- Notify your physician at the first signs of itching, redness, tiny blisters, or scaling between the toes or on the soles.

CARING FOR CORNS AND CALLUSES
- After washing feet, rub gently with a soft towel but do not tear or peel off skin.
- Do not use drugstore or home remedies for removal of corns and calluses.
- Never cut corns and calluses with a razor blade, scissors, or knife; if they are a problem, see a podiatrist.
- Wear properly fitting shoes.

FIRST AID
- Care for a cut or scratch immediately; wash the cut with soap and water; rinse well.
- Cover with a sterile gauze and paper tape (adhesive tape can irritate and tear the skin) without restricting circulation.
- Do not apply strong medicines such as iodine, boric acid, epsom salts.
- Watch for signs of infection (redness, swelling, warm feeling, pus).
- Notify physician if the injury does not get better after 24 hours or if signs of infection are present.

GENERAL
- Do not use hot water bottles or heating pads on feet.
- Do not open blisters or pick at hangnails.
- Do not soak feet because this softens skin and increases risk of infection.
- Report to physician pain, discoloration, numbness, tingling, ulcers, and any other symptoms that may develop.

- Observe for signs of infection, particularly fungal and urinary tract infection (see Chapter 6).
- Be alert to situations that can alter glucose tolerance and medication requirements (e.g., change in diet, activity, surgery, stressful situations, new medication).
- Teach proper dietary practices:
    Regular eating pattern is important.
    Change in activity alters food and medication requirement.
    Reduction and maintenance of weight within ideal range.
    Use of guides and lists (available from nutritionists) to identify nutritive content of various foods.
- Advise client to tell all health care providers with whom he/she comes in contact about diabetic condition.
- Instruct client to wear ID bracelet and carry in wallet identification card that describes condition.
- Ensure that diabetic condition is clearly noted in client's medical records.
- Administer antidiabetic medications as prescribed.
    Know that dosage is determined by weight and activity.
    Consult physician about need for dosage adjustment related to surgery, NPO status, or change in diet and/or activity.
    Review all medications administered for potential interactions (Box 5-4; Table 5-3).
- Educate client on self-injection, if required.
    Obtain special syringes/appliance to compensate for poor eyesight, arthritic joints, or other factors that could complicate injection; American Diabetes Association, occupational therapists, or rehabilitation staff may be of assistance.
    Advise about proper storage (e.g., do not keep insulin unrefrigerated more than 7 days).
    Emphasize the importance of rotating injection sites; have client record site and date injected to facilitate memory of sites used.

BOX 5-4 Oral Antidiabetic Drugs

FIRST-GENERATION AGENTS
Acetohexamide (Dymelor)
  Chlorpropamide (Chloronase, Diabinese)
  Tolazamide (Tolinase)
  Tolbutamide (Orinase, Tolbutone)

SECOND-GENERATION AGENTS
Glipizide (Glucotrol)
  Glyburide (DiaBeta, Micronase)

NURSING IMPLICATIONS
- Second-generation agents are the group of choice, because they are more potent per dose, can be administered once each day, have a shorter biologic half-life, interact with fewer drugs, and tend to be effective in reducing insulin resistance.
- Side effects can include gastrointestinal upset, anorexia, skin rash, and itching.
- Any antidiabetic medication can cause hypoglycemia; observe for signs.
- The effects of antidiabetic agents can be increased by alcohol, oral anticoagulants, isoniazid, phenylbutazone, sulfinpyrazone, and large doses of salicylates.
- Antidiabetic agents will be less effective when taken with cortisone or cortisone-like drugs, furosemide, phenytoin, thiazide diuretics, and thyroid preparations.
- Instruct client in proper administration, side effects to note and report, signs and symptoms of hypoglycemia and hyperglycemia, and importance of discussing need for dosage adjustment if there is a change in weight, activity level, or health status.

Inform client regarding importance of keeping needle sterile and how to recognize contamination.

If possible, instruct family members or close friends in technique so that they may serve as a backup, if needed.

Teach home glucose monitoring if indicated.

TABLE 5-3   Insulins

Type	Action onset (hr)	Peak (hr)	Duration (hr)
Fast-acting			
Injection, regular	1/2–1	2–3	5–8
Zine suspension: prompt, crystalline (semilente)	1	5–8	12–14
Intermediate-acting			
Globin zinc	1–2	10–18	18–24
Isophane (NPH)	1–3	10–18	18–24
Zinc (lente)	1–2	10–18	18–24
Long-acting			
Protamine zinc (PZI)	3–7	15–22	24–36
Zinc suspension (ultralente)	5–7	16–24	28–36

Nursing Implications

- Instruct client in proper administration technique; reinforce that insulin is available in various concentrations (e.g., U-40, U-100) and that the type of syringe must correspond to the concentration of insulin being used.
- Ensure that injection sites are rotated and inspected regularly.
- Be aware that although general ranges for onset, peak, and duration times are offered, individual responses can vary; observe reactions carefully, particularly during initiation of therapy.
- Teach client to recognize signs of hypoglycemia and hyperglycemia and other complications.
- Consult with physician regarding need for dosage adjustment when client is experiencing unusual stress, is having surgery, is taking new medications, or has an infection.

Hiatal hernia

GENERAL INFORMATION

The incidence of hiatal hernia increases with age and may be one of two types: *sliding hiatal hernia* and *paraesophageal hernia.* Sliding hiatal hernia is the most common type present in most older individuals and is characterized by a part of the stomach and esophagus rolling up through the diaphragm. Usually sliding hiatal hernias are asymptomatic unless reflux esophagitis occurs. Some persons may experience substernal pain and mild flatulence.

Because symptoms can mimic those associated with heart disease and other conditions, a differential diagnosis is warranted.

With paraesophageal hernia, the stomach rises alongside the esophagus, while the esophagogastric junction stays in place. In severe cases the entire stomach can rise through the diaphragm and lead to complete pyloric obstruction and gastric strangulation and perforation.

Diagnosis is confirmed by barium swallow and esophagoscopy. Many of these hernias can be successfully managed with weight reduction, a bland diet, antacids, and the elevation of the head of the bed while the client is recumbent.

CAUSATIVE/CONTRIBUTING FACTORS

Age-related degenerative changes
Weakened tissue wall between esophagus and diaphragm
Increased abdominal pressure (e.g., strain from forceful vomiting)
Obesity

CLINICAL MANIFESTATIONS

Burning pain or pressure at xiphoid process (worsened by coughing, sneezing, bending, and reclining)
Severe tightening pain
Heartburn, sour stomach
Dysphagia, belching, regurgitation, mild flatulence
Possible bleeding

ADDITIONAL NURSING INTERVENTIONS
TO INCORPORATE INTO GENERIC CARE PLAN

- Educate client regarding prescribed diet; assist in keeping a food diary and identifying eating patterns and preferences.
- Withhold food for at least 2 hours before bedtime or a nap; symptoms increase when client is in recumbent position so elevate head of bed slightly during sleep.
- Observe for and prevent aspiration; be aware that night cough can indicate that aspiration is occurring during sleep.
- Evaluate antacid therapy (Table 5-4), and observe for side effects (e.g., diarrhea, constipation, hypercalcemia, hypernatremia).
- Be alert to the possibility of myocardial infarction being present if symptoms do not subside with antacid treatment.

TABLE 5-4   Antacids

	Common side effects	Nursing implications
Aluminum hydroxide	Constipation, nausea, vomiting	Monitor serum electrolytes Advise client to take with large amounts of fluids
Calcium carbonate	Constipation, nausea, rebound hyperactivity, milk-alkali syndrome	Advise client to avoid taking with milk or foods high in vitamin D
Sodium bicarbonate	Fluid retention, belching, alkalosis, hypercalcemia, hyperphosphatemia, nausea, vomiting, headache, confusion	Caution client on sodium-restricted diet about sodium in antacid (highest sodium content: Delcid, Di-Gel, Simeco, Titralac, Trisogel)
Magnesium carbonate	Severe diarrhea	Monitor intake and output, correct diarrhea promptly

Interactions
- All antacids can decrease the effects of barbiturates, chlorpromazine, digoxin, iron prepartions, isoniazid, nitrofurantoin, oral anticoagulants, para-aminosali-cyclic acid, penicillins, phenytoin, phenylbutazone, salicylates, sulfonamides, tetracyclines, and vitamins A and C.
- Aluminum hydroxide increases the effects of meperidine, pseudoephedrine.
- Magnesium hydroxide decreases the effects of dicumarol.

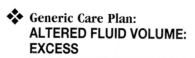

❖ **Generic Care Plan:**
  ALTERED FLUID VOLUME:
  EXCESS

GENERAL INFORMATION

Fluid volume excess is a state of vascular, cellular, or extracellular fluid overload. Additional fluids place an added burden on older hearts, which tend to be less efficient at managing such stresses. Peripheral edema is a more significant problem for the elderly because of the diminished peripheral perfusion often present; this can threaten skin integrity and promote the development of pressure ulcers. Fluid volume excess most often is manifested by edema: an accumulation of fluid in cells, tissues, or body cavities.

When edema is bilateral, cardiac problems are most likely responsible.

CAUSATIVE/CONTRIBUTING FACTORS

Decreased cardiac output (e.g., associated with congestive heart failure, myocardial infarction)
Excess fluid intake (e.g., rapid infusion of intravenous line)
Excess sodium intake
Dependent venous pooling or venostasis
Inadequate lymphatic drainage
Hormonal disturbances (e.g., pituitary, adrenal)
Steroid therapy
Liver or renal disease

CLINICAL MANIFESTATIONS (Table 5-5)

Edema
Taut, shiny skin (possibly cracked, weepy)
Weight gain
Weakness, fatigue
Shortness of breath, orthopnea
Cough
Crackles, rhonchi
Jugular venous distension
Increased blood pressure or pulse volume in affected extremity
Fluid intake exceeds output
Restlessness, anxiety

NURSING PROCESS

Assessment Considerations
- Vital signs
- Daily weight
- Record of intake and output
- Circumference of extremities and abdominal girth
- Amount of pitting at various sites
- Breath sounds, breathing pattern

Goals
- Client is free from edema.
- Client possesses balanced fluid intake and output.

TABLE 5-5   Common Fluid and Electrolyte Imbalances

Imbalance	Cause	Signs and symptoms
Dehydration	Fluid loss from vomiting, diarrhea, polyuria, excessive perspiration or drainage	Anorexia, nausea, vomiting, apathy, weakness, weight loss, postural hypotension, sunken eyes, poor skin turgor, temperature elevation, weak/rapid pulse, decreased urine output, increased specific gravity of urine, increased hematocrit
Overhydration	Congestive heart failure, cirrhosis, nephrosis, rapid infusion of intravenous fluids	Edema, ascites, effusion, dyspnea, elevated pulse, pulmonary congestion
Hyponatremia (sodium level below 135 mEq/L)	Excessive fluid intake, vomiting, gastric suctioning	Confusion, lethargy, anorexia, nausea, vomiting, seizures, coma
Hypernatremia (sodium level above 145 mEq/L)	Excessive fluid loss or inadequate fluid intake	Thirst, confusion, weakness, irritability, poor skin turgor, increased temperature, decreased urine output, increased specific gravity of urine, decreased blood pressure

Hypokalemia (potassium level below 3.4 mEq/L)	Diarrhea, vomiting, nasogastric suctioning, urinary loss, insufficient potassium intake	Weakness, irritability, anorexia, nausea, decreased reflexes, dysrhythmias
Hyperkalemia (potassium level above 5 mEq/Liter)	Acute renal failure, gastrointestinal bleeding, increased tissue injury or breakdown, acidosis	Weaknesses, paresthesias, paralysis, decreased pulse and blood pressure, cardiac arrest
Metabolic acidosis (bicarbonate level below 20 mEq/L)	Diabetic ketoacidosis, starvation, puremia, salicylate toxicity	Hyperventilation, lowered P_{CO_2}
Metabolic alkalosis (bicarbonate level above 33 mEq/L)	Vomiting, nasogastric suctioning, diuretic therapy	Depressed respirations, tetany

- Client is free from complications associated with fluid volume excess.

Nursing Interventions
- Assist with prescribed treatment to correct underlying cause.
- Strictly monitor fluid intake and output.
- Check specific gravity of urine at least daily.
- Evaluate vital signs, breath sounds, and mental status at least every 4 hours.
- Weigh daily at same time of day and with client wearing the same amount of clothing.
- If intravenous therapy is used, monitor infusion rate closely; ensure intravenous rate is not subject to positional changes.
- Change client's positions frequently; elevate edematous extremities; check skin status frequently.
- Use low semi-Fowler's position to minimize pressure on diaphragm.
- Consult with dietitian about necessary dietary modifications; restrict sodium intake, offer salt substitutes if appropriate.
- Provide good skin care.
- If client is taking diuretics, monitor output carefully, ensure bathroom facilities are easily available.
- Avoid rapid mobilization of severe edema (profound intoxication can occur from the metabolic debris carried in the fluids).
- Monitor diuretics and other therapies carefully for desired results, possible complications.

Evaluation
- Client possesses normal fluid and electrolyte levels.
- Client resumes normal weight.
- Client is free from edema.
- Client is free from complications associated with fluid volume excess.

Possible Related Nursing Diagnoses
Activity intolerance, high risk for
Altered tissue perfusion
Fatigue
Impaired skin integrity, high risk for
Infection, high risk for

❖ Generic Care Plan:
FLUID VOLUME DEFICIT

GENERAL INFORMATION

A reduction in vascular, cellular, or intracellular fluid is a fluid volume deficit. Older adults are at high risk for dehydration because of age-related changes, such as reduced intracellular fluid and decreased thirst sensation. Some elderly persons have health problems that interfere with their ability to request, obtain, and ingest an adequate amount of fluid.

CAUSATIVE/CONTRIBUTING FACTORS

Excess fluid loss (e.g., polyuria, excessive wound drainage, diarrhea, vomiting)
Inadequate fluid intake (e.g., unable to reach fluids; oral pain; swallowing disorder; altered cognition, level of consciousness, or mood)
Increased metabolic rate (e.g., fever)
Medications (diuretics, laxatives, sedatives)

CLINICAL MANIFESTATIONS

Delirium
Lethargy, lightheadedness
Dryness of lips, oral mucosa, conjunctiva
Poor skin turgor
Nausea, anorexia
Shrunken, furrowed tongue (usually develops in late stage)
Increased temperature
Increased pulse
Decreased blood pressure
Decreased or excessive urine output
Fluid output exceeds intake, concentrated urine
Weight loss

NURSING PROCESS

Assessment Considerations
- Vital signs
- Weight

- Mental status
- Fluid intake and output
- Urinalysis (specific gravity greater than 1.030, urine choline below 50 mEq)
- Electrolytes; elevated BUN, sodium; possible rise in hematocrit

Goals
- Client possesses fluid and electrolyte levels within normal range.
- Client ingests at least 2000 ml of fluids daily.

Nursing Interventions
- Offer fluids regularly to prevent dehydration; use alternate sources such as ices, Jell-O, citrus fruits; ensure approximately 2000 ml of fluid daily unless otherwise contraindicated.
- Identify persons at high risk for dehydration (e.g., those who are confused, depressed, tube fed, immobile, anorexic, fatigued, vomiting, or taking sedatives, tranquilizers, diuretics, laxatives); take appropriate actions.
- Replace fluids as prescribed; space them over 24 hours; avoid fluid overload by monitoring for adequate output.

Evaluation
- Client's laboratory test results demonstrate fluids and electrolytes within normal ranges.
- Client is free from signs of dehydration.
- Client consumes at least 2000 ml of fluids per day.
- Client's intake and output are balanced.

Possible Related Nursing Diagnoses
Activity intolerance
Altered nutrition: less than body requirements
Altered oral mucous membrane
Altered thought processes
Diarrhea
Fatigue
Impaired skin integrity, high risk for
Incontinence
Infection, high risk for

❖ Generic Care Plan:
IMPAIRED SKIN INTEGRITY

Impaired skin integrity is a state in which there is disruption to the healthy, normal status of the skin. This can be *potential impaired skin integrity,* in which there is a risk to the healthy status of the skin, or *actual impaired skin integrity,* in which an alteration to the skin's status exists.

Skin changes in the elderly cause them to be highly vulnerable to skin impairment and slower healing when skin injury does occur. Such skin changes include the following:

- Dryness, atrophy of sweat glands, decreased perspiration
- Loss of turgor and elasticity
- Hair loss, dryness, and graying
- Reduced vascularity, capillary fragility, and easy bruising
- Flattening of papillae of epidermis
- Thinning of dermal area; loss of strength and elasticity of dermis
- Loss of subcutaneous fat
- Lentigo senilis ("age spots") on skin exposed to sunlight

Careful attention to the older client's appetite, nutritional status, hygienic practices, continence, skin condition, and energy and activity levels is necessary to identify potential problems that could threaten skin integrity.

Good fluid intake and a balanced diet promote healthy skin. Vitamin A helps maintain the keratin layer of the epidermis, and niacin and riboflavin help to prevent dermatitis. Vitamin C assists in collagen synthesis; zinc and iron promote skin integrity and healing.

Common geriatric skin problems are seborrheic dermatitis and seborrheic keratosis. The former is characterized by loose scaling on the scalp, eyebrows, axillae and anogenital area, behind the ears, and under the breasts. The latter is a benign wartlike lesion that first appears as yellow plaque covered with oily-looking scales that may become pigmented later.

CAUSATIVE/CONTRIBUTING FACTORS

Advanced age
Mobility deficit; immobility

Altered circulation; peripheral vascular disease
General debilitation
Infections
Metabolic or endocrine disorders (e.g., diabetes mellitus)
Altered nutritional state (e.g., emaciation, obesity, dehydration)
Incontinence
Mechanical factors (e.g., shearing forces, restraints, traction)
Altered sensations (e.g., decreased ability to sense pressure, pain)
Trauma, surgery, radiation
Moist, closed environments (e.g., skinfolds, perianal area)
Unprotected exposure to sunlight
Use of harsh soaps or topical products
Allergic reaction

CLINICAL MANIFESTATIONS

Denuded skin
Erythema
Lesions
Pruritus
Pressure areas or ulcers
Pain or numbness
Stomas or fistulas
Burns
Edema
Irritation
Senile purpura

NURSING PROCESS

Assessment Considerations
- Skin color, moisture, turgor, integrity
- Presence of rashes, discolorations, ulcers, scratches, lesions, other abnormalities
- History of risk factors
- Symptoms: itching, burning, discomfort
- Review of normal hygienic practices: skin care practices, cosmetic use
- Diet
- General health status, activity pattern

Goals
- Client maintains intact skin.
- Client restores skin integrity.
- Client experiences a reduction in size of skin lesion.
- Client is free from signs of impaired skin integrity.

Nursing Interventions
- Assist with identification and treatment of underlying cause.
- Evaluate client's risk of impaired skin integrity; implement measures specific to risk factors.
- Inspect client's entire skin surface for signs of skin impairment.
- Offer a diet high in protein, carbohydrate, vitamins, and minerals (unless contraindicated); consult with nutritionist as necessary.
- Evaluate client's need for position change and change position accordingly: For some clients, pressure may develop within 2 hours, so a turning schedule of every 2 hours is insufficient to prevent skin breakdown. Initially, assess pressure points after client has been in a position for ½ hour; if no signs of pressure are present allow client to remain in position for 1 hour and check for signs of pressure; if no pressure is present allow client to remain in position for 1½ hours and check for signs of pressure. Any sign of pressure detected at any time interval indicates that the time interval is the maximum length of time that client can be in that position.
- Ensure that clients who are in sitting positions have frequent position changes.
- Avoid shearing force by not elevating bed more than 30 degrees and not pulling client across or up in bed.
- Use pillows for positioning and support to prevent skin surfaces from touching each other and to provide air circulation when client is totally immobile.
- Avoid excessive dryness of skin by limiting bathing to approximately twice per week; give daily partial baths to high odor areas.
- Use mild, nonirritating soap; apply moisturizers to skin after bathing.
- Keep skin clean and dry; blot, do not rub older skin.
- Inspect moist, hidden areas regularly, particularly the scalp, between the toes, axillae, undersurface of breast, and anal and genital areas.

- Pad potential breakdown sites with sheepskin or Gelfoam, or use alternating pressure mattresses and water beds if client is immobile; use heel and elbow protectors, foot cradle, and cushions on wheelchairs.
- Keep sheets and pads dry and wrinkle free; examine the bed or chair for foreign objects.
- Massage bony prominences regularly; promote circulation by giving whirlpool and range of motion (ROM) exercises on a regular basis.
- Pay particular attention to keeping the incontinent client clean and dry; use effective adult briefs, and cleanse client with each change.
- Advise client not to scratch or rub skin or apply irritating or drying substances.
- Administer medications as ordered (e.g., antihistamines, ointments).
- Promote touch; educate family members/visitors about realities of skin disorder and ability to have direct contact with client.
- Assist client in achieving positive appearance.
- Instruct persons of all ages to protect skin when exposed to sunlight.

Evaluation
- Client is free from impairments of skin integrity.
- Client demonstrates appropriate skin care techniques.
- Client's lesions are reduced in size or healed.

Possible Related Nursing Diagnoses
Altered nutrition
Altered thought processes
Diarrhea
Disturbance in body image
Fluid volume deficit
Hyperthermia
Hypothermia
Impaired physical mobility
Incontinence
Infection, high risk for
Pain
Self-care deficit: bathing, toileting, feeding, moving
Sensory/perceptual alteration: tactile

❖❖ Selected Health Problem Associated with IMPAIRED SKIN INTEGRITY
Pressure ulcer

GENERAL INFORMATION

Pressure ulcers, areas of necrosis of the skin and subcutaneous tissue caused by insufficient circulation secondary to pressure, are a major risk to the elderly that can threaten function and life. Common sites for pressure ulcer formation are over bony prominences that are not padded well with subcutaneous fat, such as the sacrum, greater trochanter, ischial tuberosities, elbows, and heels. The ulcers can be superficial (confined to the outermost layers of the skin) or deep (damage to all layers of the skin and possibly muscle and bone).

Open sores extend from the surface downward and have a wide diameter. *Closed sores* originate in underlying tissue and extend to the surface, with only a small ulcer being visible. Signs of infection may be present such as *Pseudomonas,* a frequently cultured organism characterized by green or blue-green purulent drainage.

Pressure ulcers progress through several phases in their development:

Hyperemia: Localized redness; disappears when pressure is removed and tissue circulation restored

Ischemia: Discoloration and swelling of skin; occurs after 6 or more hours of continuous pressure or sooner in a debilitated person

Ulceration: Open lesion exposing subcutaneous tissue

Necrosis: Dead skin that may extend through fascia and bone; eschar often is present

The Omnibus Budget Reconciliation Act (OBRA) that brought dramatic reform to nursing home practice included a requirement for a standardized assessment of all residents of long-term care facilities. One of the outgrowths of this effort was an assessment tool that included specific criteria for staging pressure ulcers (Figure 5-1)

Stage 1: A persistent area of skin redness (without a break in the skin) that does not disappear when pressure is relieved

Stage 2: A partial-thickness loss of skin layers that presents clinically as an abrasion, blister, or shallow crater

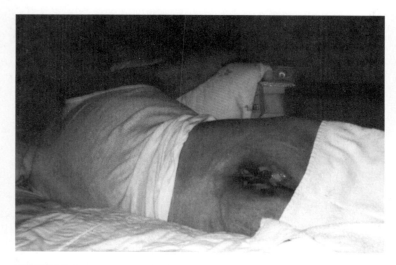

FIGURE 5-1 Pressure ulcer located on the client's tailbone or coccyx. It is classified as stage 3 because it involves muscle tissue. (From Castillo HM: *The nurse assistant in long-term care: a rehabilitative approach,* St Louis, 1992, Mosby–Year Book)

Stage 3: A full-thickness loss of skin, exposing the subcutaneous tissues; presents as a deep crater with or without undermining adjacent tissue

Stage 4: A full-thickness loss of skin and subcutaneous tissue, exposing muscle and/or bone

The use of this staging system in all practice sites can assist in improved communication regarding the status of pressure ulcers.

CAUSATIVE/CONTRIBUTING FACTORS

Prolonged pressure against bony prominence leading to tissue anoxia and ischemia

Shearing force: sitting up in bed, being pulled across bed

Incontinence

Debilitated state

Immobility

Reduced sensations for pain and pressure

Medications that decrease sensitivity, alertness, or mobility

Vitamin C deficiency, hypoproteinemia, anemia

ADDITIONAL NURSING INTERVENTIONS
TO INCORPORATE INTO GENERIC CARE PLAN

- Determine cause, type, and stage of ulcer.
- Follow prescribed treatment plan (Box 5-5).
- Position client off affected area.
- Obtain special beds, mattresses, pads, protectors as appropriate.
- Keep dressings clean and intact.
- Ensure good nutritional state; consult with physician and nutritionist regarding protein and vitamin supplements.
- Monitor healing progress; measure and document diameter and depth of ulcer daily.
- Observe for signs of infection; if symptoms are present, culture the ulcer.

BOX 5-5   Treatments Used for Pressure Ulcers

TRANSPARENT, VAPOR-PERMEABLE DRESSINGS
- These are polyurethane dressings that allow gases (e.g., oxygen) to be exchanged but not fluids. This prevents potentially contaminating fluids from entering the ulcer and allows the ulcer to have an environment that promotes healing.
- Dressing should not be tight since this can cause a shearing force.
- Dressing should cover area about 1 inch beyond ulcer.
- Dressings usually are left in place 5 to 7 days.
- Exudate varies in color and consistency and should not be drained. Excessive exudate that drains from edge of dressing is cause for dressing change.
- Change the dressing if infection is suspected.
- Examples include Biocclusive, Tegaderm, and Op-Site.

OCCLUSIVE BARRIERS
- These are dressings that contain absorbent hydrocolloid particles that expand and form a moist gel when they come in contact with wound drainage to form a closed, moist environment.
- The surrounding skin must be clean and dry for the dressing to adhere.
- The dressing should extend at least $1\frac{1}{2}$ inches beyond the edge of the ulcer.
- Dressings usually are left in place 5 to 7 days unless leakage occurs.
- These dressings are not recommended for ulcers showing any clinical signs of infection.
- Examples include DuoDerm and Comfeel Ulcus.

Continued.

BOX 5-5   Treatments Used for Pressure Ulcers—cont'd

LIQUID BARRIERS
- These agents are applied via spray, roll-on, or wipe-on and form a waterproof coating over an area. This coating offers protection against maceration and shearing.
- Water will not penetrate or remove these agents although soap solutions will.
- Examples include Bard Protective Barrier Film and United Skin Prep.

CHEMICAL DEBRIDEMENT
- Debriding enzymes are used to remove superficial layers of dead tissue; however, they will not penetrate eschar. Eschar must be mechanically or surgically debrided.
- These agents can be inhibited by the use of topical antibacterials and antiseptics.
- Examples include Elase and Travase.

MECHANICAL DEBRIDEMENT
- This method attempts to remove necrotic tissue and drainage through the use of wet-to-dry dressings or irrigations.
- Wet-to-dry dressings usually are changed every shift.
- This is not an effective means to remove eschar.

SURGICAL DEBRIDEMENT
- This is the most effective means of removing infected or necrotic tissue.
- Skin grafts or flaps may be used to close the area. Pressure should be kept off the area.
- Postoperatively, observations should be made for infection and hemorrhage.
- CO_2 lasers may be used as a painless means to quickly debride an ulcer. This method sterilizes the ulcer and stimulates the release of growth factors that promote healing.

GENERAL MEASURES
- Keep wound clean. Cleansing may be done with normal saline solution or the use of a mild antibacterial solution followed by a normal saline rinse.
- Keep dressings clean; change if they become soiled.
- Keep area dry enough for dressing to adhere.
- Avoid the use of heating lamps; in addition to risk of burn injury, they can dehydrate wounds and interfere with healing.
- Ensure client ingests adequate diet; consult with nutritionist and physician regarding need for supplements.
- Observe for signs of infection and related complications
- Monitor healing progress; measure depth and diameter of ulcer and observe color and characteristics of drainage.

❖ Generic Care Plan:
ALTERED ORAL MUCOUS MEMBRANE

GENERAL INFORMATION

Altered oral mucous membrane is an interruption in the integrity of the layers and/or protective properties of the oral mucosa. Older adults are at risk for this problem because of age-related dryness of the oral cavity and the high prevalence of periodontal disease and poor dental status.

Health status of the oral cavity has a significant impact on dietary intake, self-image, speech and communication, socialization, and general health.

CAUSATIVE/CONTRIBUTING FACTORS

Advanced age: reduced saliva production; atrophy of the mucosal epithelium, which increases the risk of irritation and infection
Poor-fitting dentures
Poor dental status: periodontal disease, broken teeth
Medications: anticholinergics, antibiotics, chemotherapeutic agents
Years of smoking, drinking irritating liquids
Burns from excessively hot food or drink
Disease: cancer, anemia, infections
Malnourishment
Limited ability to floss, brush, or clean dentures

CLINICAL MANIFESTATIONS

Lips: fissures, lesions, ulcers, discoloration, dryness, asymmetry
Tongue: ulcers, unusually raised papillae, fissures, smoothness, pain, coating, white patchy areas, masses, limited movement
Gums and mucous membrane: ulcers, fissures, white patchy areas, masses, discoloration, swelling, numbness, bleeding, friction rubs from teeth or dentures
Teeth: decay, brittleness, looseness, jagged edges, poor hygiene
Dentures: looseness, broken teeth, rough surface, poor hygiene
Decreased salivation
Pain
Decreased appetite, weight loss

NURSING PROCESS

Assessment Considerations
- History of symptoms
- Condition of oral cavity (including tissue beneath dentures)
- Condition of teeth, gums
- Fit, condition, cleanliness of dentures
- Pattern of oral hygiene; self-care capacity
- Medications being used
- Diseases possessed
- Symptoms: pain, halitosis, bleeding

Goals
- Client demonstrates good oral hygiene practices.
- Client possesses healthy gums, teeth, lips, and tongue.
- Client ingests a well-balanced diet and is free from nutritional problems associated with impaired mucous membrane.

Nursing Interventions
- Instruct client in good oral hygiene measures (Figure 5-2) (Box 5-6).
- Advise client that water jet sprays are not recommended for older adults with oral infections, because they can spray bacteria onto unhealthy gums, leading to serious infection.

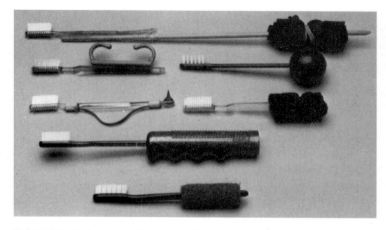

FIGURE 5-2 Adaptive aids for brushing can promote independence in oral hygiene. (From Papas AS, Niessen LC, Chauncey HH: *Geriatric dentistry: aging and oral health*, St Louis, 1991, Mosby–Year Book.)

BOX 5-6   Assisting Clients with Oral Hygiene

Nursing staff are in an ideal position to evaluate clients' oral health and identify problems of the oral cavity. No other discipline has regular, direct contact with client's oral cavities as does the nursing staff. Good oral hygiene and prompt identification and treatment of oral health problems can make a tremendous difference in the physical, emotional, and social well-being of clients.

BRUSHING

It is the action of the toothbrush, not the toothpaste, that removes plaque from teeth. A proper toothbrush has stiff, soft bristles.

Use a systematic, consistent approach to brushing. Begin brushing the back teeth. These teeth can be easier to reach if the mouth is opened slightly rather than wide open. Hold the brush horizontally and tilt at a 45-degree angle with the teeth. Use short strokes to brush back and forth with light pressure for about 10 seconds. Continue moving to all tooth surfaces. Be sure to brush the gums near the teeth to stimulate the gum and remove plaque from the sulcus. Brushing the tongue helps to reduce mouth odors and refreshes the mouth.

The teeth should be brushed at least once in the morning and at night.

Toothpaste isn't necessary for brushing although it helps to carry away loosened plaque and debris, and it leaves the mouth feeling fresh. Also, the fluoride in toothpaste helps to strengthen tooth enamel from decay.

Electric toothbrushes and toothbrushes with modified handles can aid persons who need special assistance with brushing; dental health professionals and occupational therapists can assist in locating special equipment for oral hygiene.

FLOSSING

Brushing cannot reach all tooth surfaces or adequately reach the sulcus, so flossing is necessary to loosen plaque from these areas.

Any type of floss will be effective. Cut about 18 inches and wrap the ends around your fingers so that 5 to 6 inches remain. Holding the floss taut, place the floss behind the last tooth in the rear of the mouth and insert until it touches the gum. Rub the floss up and down the tooth (not back and forth) several times. Go to the next tooth and repeat. Use a systematic approach to ensure all teeth are flossed. If the floss becomes frayed or covered with plaque, unwind a fresh section and wrap the used one on your finger. If bleeding or pain results, too much pressure is being exerted. Rinse the mouth after all teeth have been flossed.

Floss holders and floss threaders can be useful aids for persons unable to manipulate floss with their fingers or who do not have the use of both hands.

Continued.

BOX 5-6   Assisting Clients with Oral Hygiene—cont'd

INTERDENTAL STIMULATORS

Interdental stimulators, or gum massagers, come in the form of soft wooden sticks, and rubber or plastic cones. They are effective in loosening plaque in areas not reached by brushing and flossing.

Interdental stimulators are less useful in older persons because the elderly tend to have a large space between their teeth and gum lines. For these individuals, the use of an interproximal brush (shaped like a miniature baby bottle brush) is effective in loosening plaque from the sulcus.

DENTURE CARE

Dentures need daily brushing to prevent plaque buildup; commercial denture cleaners or soap and water can aid in keeping dentures clean. (Cleanse dentures over a basin of water or washcloth to cushion and prevent damage, should the dentures accidentally be dropped.) The mouth should be rinsed after every meal to remove debris.

Denture adhesives can be helpful in keeping dentures in place. All old adhesive should be removed from the dentures during cleansing.

The gums should be stimulated and cleansed through daily brushing.

Any remaining teeth need routine tooth care.

While the dentures are removed for cleaning, the oral cavity should be inspected for irritation, sores, and other problems. Dentures should be kept in a moist environment (e.g., water) to prevent warping if they are removed for a prolonged time.

Poor-fitting, warped, or broken dentures should be replaced or repaired.

GENERAL MEASURES

Use lip balm or petroleum jelly to prevent cracking of the lips.

Motivate clients to be attentive to oral hygiene and recognize their efforts when they are.

From Eliopoulos C: Oral health, *Long-Term Care Edu* 3 (lesson 7), 1992.

- Suggest that client have name or social security number engraved on dentures to serve as a means of identification.

Evaluation
- Client possesses healthy oral mucosa.
- Client demonstrates appropriate oral hygiene practices.

Possible Related Nursing Diagnoses
Altered nutrition
Disturbance in body image

Infection, high risk for
Knowledge deficit
Pain
Self-care deficit: hygiene
Sensory-perceptual alteration: taste

RECOMMENDED READINGS

Bergstrom N, Braden BJ, Laguzza A et al: The Braden scale for predicting pressure sore risk, *Nurs Res* 36:205, 1987.
Braden BJ, Bryant R: Innovations to prevent and treat pressure ulcers. *Geriatr Nurs* 11(4):182, 1990.
Davidson MB: Carbohydrate metabolism and diabetes mellitus. In Abrams WB, Berkow R, editors: *The Merck manual of geriatrics,* Rahway, NJ, 1990, Merck Sharp and Dohme Research Laboratories.
Diabetic update 93, *Nurs 93,* pp 59-61, Aug 1993.
Macheca MK: Diabetic hypoglycemia: keeping the threat at bay, *Am J Nurs* 93(4):26-30, 1993.
Morley JE: Anorexia in older patients: its meaning and management, *Geriatrics* 45(12):59, 1990.
Pajk M: Pressure sores. In Abrams WB, Berkow R, editors: *The Merck manual of geriatrics,* Rahway, NJ, 1990, Merck Sharp and Dohme Research Laboratories.
Yen PK: Following the diabetic diet, *Geriatr Nurs* 11(6):303, 1990.
Yen PK: The picture of malnutrition, *Geriatr Nurs* 10(3):159, 1989.

6

Elimination

Elimination problems, common among the elderly, provoke anxiety and distress for both the client and the nurse. Many factors contribute to these problems in old age.

The risk of constipation increases because of slower peristalsis, the tendency to consume less bulk and fluids, reduced activity levels, and diminished nerve sensation to the lower bowel that reduces the signal of needing to defecate. Reduced bladder capacity can increase the frequency of urination, and weaker muscles along the urinary tract can create problems with urinary retention, dribbling, and stress incontinence. An enlarged prostate gland, urinary tract infections, calculi, altered mental status, and other disorders that are more prevalent in the older population can promote incontinence. Medications can impact bowel and bladder elimination in a variety of ways ranging from urinary retention to constipation. Toileting habits, environmental factors, and functional capacity also contribute to elimination problems.

Older persons lose dignity and self-esteem when they have difficulty controlling their body functions not to mention the risks to comfort, skin integrity, and general well-being. An essential nursing role is to facilitate the maintenance and, as necessary and possible, reestablishment of normal elimination patterns.

❖ Generic Care Plan:
CONSTIPATION

GENERAL INFORMATION

Constipation is the abnormal delay or infrequent passage of dry, hardened feces and is one of the most common health problems for the elderly. The colon can lose innervation and experience smooth muscle atrophy.

CAUSATIVE/CONTRIBUTING FACTORS

Inactivity, decrease in activity level
Poor bowel habits
    Not establishing regular pattern or time
    Ignoring signal for elimination
Poor nutrition
    Decreased appetite
    Poor oral health
    Inadequate intake of bulk
    Inadequate consumption of fluid
Emotional problems
    Reduced food intake and inactivity secondary to depression, boredom, grief
    Anorexia secondary to emotional disturbance
Socioeconomic factors
    Inadequate income to purchase proper food
    Inability to store or prepare proper food
    Self-imposed fluid restrictions to avoid urinary frequency
Medications
    Iron preparations
    Antihypertensives
    Analgesics
    Tranquilizers
    Anticholinergics
    Antacids containing calcium carbonate
    Laxatives (excessive use can cause muscular atony, decreased awareness of presence of stool)
Organic problems
    Hypothyroidism
    Tumors
    Diabetic neuropathy

Anorectal lesions, hemorrhoids
Colon stricture
Decreased gastrointestinal motility
Dementia
Hypokalemia
Hypercalcemia

CLINICAL MANIFESTATIONS

Difficult passage of hard, dry stool
Decreased frequency of bowel movements
Abdominal fullness, discomfort, distension
Rectal fullness, pressure
Flatulence
Presence of hard stool in rectum on palpation
Nausea, vomiting, anorexia
Headache, lethargy
Decreased activity

NURSING PROCESS

Assessment Considerations

- History of pattern and characteristics of bowel movements (have client keep record of elimination pattern)
- Review of dietary habits, recent food intake, activity pattern
- Review of all prescription and over-the-counter drugs consumed
- Client's definition of constipation (many older adults interpret lack of a daily bowel movement as constipation, despite the absence of clinical signs)
- History of recent losses, changes, or events that could impact physical or emotional status, such as retirement, death of a loved one, recent period of bed rest, new medical disorder, family problems
- Auscultate bowel sounds; palpate abdomen and rectum
- Note character and frequency of stools
- Presence of other signs and symptoms
    Alternating constipation and diarrhea (tumors, irritable colon, fecal impaction)
    Nausea, vomiting (diverticulitis, bowel obstruction)
    Low back pain (irritable colon)
    Rectal pain, fissures

Thin stools (diverticular disease, irritable colon, hemorrhoids, rectal cancer)

Intolerance to cold, weight gain, hoarseness, slower mental function (hypothyroidism)

Bloody stools (hemorrhoids, ulcerative colitis, diverticulitis, impaction, colon cancer)

Goals
- Client develops regular pattern of bowel elimination.
- Client learns ways to prevent constipation and appropriate interventions to alleviate constipation.

Nursing Interventions
- Ensure treatment of underlying condition or disease that promotes constipation (e.g., depression, hemorrhoids).
- Encourage changes in dietary habit such as the following:
    Increase dietary fiber and bulk (bran, whole grains, raw vegetables and fruit).
    Introduce foods that may induce elimination (prunes, chocolate, spinach).
    Ask client to identify foods that have produced loose stools in the past and incorporate them into diet in moderation.
    Increase fluid intake unless contraindicated.
- Increase general activity level and encourage daily exercise.
- Teach client to develop good bowel habits, such as attending to physiologic cues and toileting regularly at times when success is most likely (e.g., after breakfast when the introduction of food following nighttime inactivity stimulates the gastrointestinal tract).
- Administer laxatives as prescribed (see Table 6-1); instruct client in safe laxative use; wean from laxatives and enemas if indicated and if muscle tone is adequate.
- Review medications to determine those that can promote constipation; consult with physician regarding change in medications if possible.
- Be aware that the older client may be unable to fully empty bowel at one sitting.
    Have client toilet 30 to 45 minutes after the first bowel movement to encourage completion of bowel elimination.
    Alert staff to take requests for second toileting seriously.
- Provide privacy and time alone to defecate.

- Avoid using a bedpan if at all possible with a bed-bound client because it forces the extension of the legs, abdominal hyper-extension, and defecation without muscular help, thereby causing undue strain; if the client is not properly positioned, gravity cannot assist the passage of stool.
- Use a commode chair or toilet with the able client to promote relaxation.
- Teach techniques to facilitate elimination.
    Elevate feet slightly using small footrest or book.
    Lean forward to increase abdominal pressure.
- Remember straining and enemas can stimulate the vagus nerve and inhibit heart function because of the Valsalva maneuver.

Evaluation
- Client regularly passes formed stool with no or minimal discomfort.
- Client has bowel movements without inducement by laxatives, suppositories, or enemas.

Possible Related Nursing Diagnoses
Altered nutrition: less than body requirements
Bowel incontinence
Diarrhea
Self-care deficit: toileting

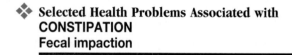

❖ Selected Health Problems Associated with CONSTIPATION
Fecal impaction

GENERAL INFORMATION

Fecal impaction is a large accumulation of feces in the rectum or colon that is difficult to move. It is the most common reason for nonacute intestinal obstruction. Colorectal cancer and cardiac disease are relative contraindications to manually removing an impaction.

CAUSATIVE/CONTRIBUTING FACTORS

Irregular evacuation pattern
Dehydration

Decreased motility of gastrointestinal tract
Colorectal disease
Impaired mental function
Painful defecation (e.g., related to anal fissures, hemorrhoids)
Sensorimotor disorders (e.g., cerebrovascular accident [CVA], neurologic disease)
Side effects of drugs (antacids, iron, barium, aluminum, calcium)
Stress
Lack of privacy for toileting

CLINICAL MANIFESTATIONS

Absence of regular bowel movement
Abdominal fullness and discomfort
Oozing of fecal material from rectum (sometimes resembling diarrhea)
Elevated temperature
Poor appetite
Lethargy
Restlessness
Fecal mass palpable on digital examination

ADDITIONAL NURSING INTERVENTIONS
TO INCORPORATE INTO GENERIC CARE PLAN

- Prepare client for removal of fecal impaction:
    Explain procedure.
    Position client on left side with knees flexed; drape appropriately.
    Ask client to take deep breaths to diminish effects of Valsalva maneuver.
- Remove impaction (if ordered and consistent with agency or facility policy):
    Insert lubricated, gloved finger into rectum using a circular motion; remove small masses.
    If mass is large, insert two lubricated, gloved fingers and break up mass before removing.
    Talk with client throughout procedure; promote relaxation.
- Use other measures, as necessary:
    Use warm, oil retention enemas (unless contraindicated).
    Use hydrogen peroxide (50 to 100 ml through a rectal tube) unless bowel disease is present or client has had recent surgery to area.

- Record results, client's tolerance, and any problems noted.
- Observe for signs of obstruction.
- Institute measures to prevent recurrence; monitor bowel elimination pattern.

Hemorrhoids

GENERAL INFORMATION

A hemorrhoid is a mass of dilated veins in swollen tissue situated near the anal sphincter. Internal hemorrhoids arise above the anorectal line; external hemorrhoids arise below and are visible on inspection. Hemorrhoids can develop in old age or be a chronic problem from earlier years.

CAUSATIVE/CONTRIBUTING FACTORS

Chronic constipation
Heavy lifting
Straining while defecating
Long periods of standing or sitting
Obesity
Portal hypertension

CLINICAL MANIFESTATIONS

Anal itching
Bleeding during or after bowel movements
Pain
Bulge in rectal area
Swollen, dilated perianal veins

ADDITIONAL NURSING INTERVENTIONS
TO INCORPORATE INTO GENERIC CARE PLAN

- Teach dietary modifications (low residue, high fiber) to prevent constipation.
- Administer and instruct client in safe use of stool softeners/ laxatives (Table 6-1).

TABLE 6-1 Laxatives

Categories	Examples	Action	Nursing implications
Bulk formers	Methylcellulose Psyllium	Absorb water in intestines and expand, creating more bulk; extra bulk distends intestines and increases peristalsis	Good fluid intake necessary to prevent intestinal obstruction. Effects *usually* noted in 12-24 hr. Do not use when intestinal obstruction, abdominal pain, dehydration, nausea, or vomiting is suspected or present; not absorbed systemically.
Stool softeners	Docusate calcium Docusate sodium	Promote collection of fluid in stool, creating a softer stool mass and easier bowel movements	Carefully evaluate use with clients who have cardiac, renal, or other problems impairing management of excess fluid. Effects usually noted in 24-28 hr. Do not stimulate peristalsis: more effective as prevention rather than cure; absorbed systemically.
Hyperosmolar agents	Glycerin Magnesium salts Saline	Pull fluid into colon (salt-based laxatives also draw fluid to small intestine), causing bowel distension, increased peristalsis	Glycerin is administered as suppository or enema; can cause cramps. Ensure good fluid intake with administration of magnesium salts. Effects usually noted within 1-3 hr.

Continued.

TABLE 6-1   Laxatives—cont'd

Categories	Examples	Action	Nursing implications
			Avoid magnesium salts in clients with abdominal pain, serious cardiac problems, renal disease, intestinal obstruction, nausea, vomiting, or fecal impaction. Do not administer *any* medication 2 hr before or after saline laxative because saline interferes with absorption. Magnesium salts are absorbed systematically; if used on a long-term basis, periodically evaluate serum electrolytes.
Stimulants	Cascara sagrada Senna	Irritate smooth muscle of intestine to increase peristalsis; draw fluid into small intestine and colon to distend bowel, further increasing peristalsis	Use on short-term basis only; long-term use can cause electrolyte imbalance, particularly hypokalemia. Effects are usually noted within 6-10 hr (senna is more potent than cascara). Cascara can discolor urine (advise patient). Avoid use in clients with nausea, vomiting, intestinal obstruction, abdominal pain, or fecal impaction;

TABLE 6-1 Laxatives—cont'd

Categories	Examples	Action	Nursing implications
			some systematic absorption.
Lubricants	Mineral oil	Coats fecal matter and prevents absorption of fluid from feces, resulting in easier passage of stool	Avoid use in clients with nausea, vomiting, intestinal obstruction, abdominal pain, or fecal impaction.
			Administer on an empty stomach, since it will delay emptying. Effects are usually noted within 6-8 hr.
			Minimize unpleasant taste by having patient hold ice chips on tongue before administration or by mixing with soda or juice; not recommended for older persons because of serious complications that can result in:
			• Dehydration from diarrhea
			• Lipid pneumonias and lung abscesses from aspiration
			• Deficiencies of fat-soluble vitamins A, D, K, and E (dissolved in and excreted with the oil
			• Emulsified oil is absorbed more completely than nonemulsified.

- Relieve discomfort and pain with warm sitz baths.
    Measure water temperature carefully since the elderly are more susceptible to burns.
    Observe for dizziness caused by lowered blood pressure (blood is pulled to lower extremities during sitz bath).
- Teach avoidance of straining and sitting on toilet for long periods and care of anal area with compresses and ointments.
- Prepare client for surgery if a hemorroidectomy is recommended.

Diverticular disease

GENERAL INFORMATION

Diverticulosis is a condition in which multiple pouches form along the intestinal wall. Diverticula are most common in the sigmoid area and occur more in women than men. They usually develop in the fifth decade of life and increase in size and number with time if untreated. Diverticulitis is inflammation of the diverticula.

CAUSATIVE/CONTRIBUTING FACTORS

Obesity
Low-residue diet
Chronic constipation
Genetic predisposition

CLINICAL MANIFESTATIONS

Diverticulosis usually asymptomatic
Diverticulitis
    Lower left quadrant pain and cramps; tenderness of area on palpation
    Flatulence
    Nausea and vomiting
    Fever
    Bowel irregularity
    Change in bowel habits (diarrhea, constipation, or both)

Periodic urgency of colon evacuation
Blood in stool

ADDITIONAL NURSING INTERVENTIONS TO INCORPORATE INTO GENERIC CARE PLAN

- Relieve pain (see Chapter 8).
- Teach diet modification (high fiber, low residue) and restriction of foods known to aggravate condition.
- Prevent diverticulitis (see Chapter 4).
- Administer antibiotics as ordered (see Box 4-1).
- Teach client how to avoid intraabdominal pressure by avoiding straining at stool, vomiting, lifting, and restrictive clothing.
- Prepare client for surgical intervention (colon resection) if recommended.

Colorectal cancer

GENERAL INFORMATION

Colorectal cancer refers to a malignant neoplasm originating in the colon or rectum. It is the second most common malignancy in the United States. The incidence of colorectal cancer begins to increase significantly after 40 years of age and peaks in the eighth decade of life. It affects both sexes equally. Most cancers of the large intestine occur in the descending colon, rectosigmoid, or rectum. Cancer occurring in the ascending colon may have different clinical manifestations from that occurring in the descending colon.

CAUSATIVE/CONTRIBUTING FACTORS

Advanced age
Familial polyposis; chronic ulcerative colitis
Higher incidence with:
> Diet low in fiber and high in refined carbohydrates and animal fat
> Higher socioeconomic groups
> Persons with history of breast cancer, inflammatory bowel disease, chronic parasitic infections

CLINICAL MANIFESTATIONS

Asymptomatic in early stage (emphasizes importance of routine proctosigmoidoscopic examination or stool testing for occult blood)

Left-sided mass (descending colon)
>   Weight loss
>   Narrow, ribbonlike stools
>   Rectal bleeding
>   Cramping abdominal pain
>   Rectal mass
>   Mucous discharge
>   Changes in bowel habit

Right-sided mass (ascending colon)
>   Usually asymptomatic
>   Weakness and fatigue
>   Occult bleeding
>   Diarrhea
>   Palpable mass
>   Iron deficiency anemia
>   Complaints of vague abdominal pain

ADDITIONAL NURSING INTERVENTIONS
TO INCORPORATE INTO GENERIC CARE PLAN

- Support treatment plan:
>   Radiation and chemotherapy (palliative treatment to shrink tumor)
>   Surgery
>   Ascending colon: right colectomy with ileotransverse anastomosis
>   Descending colon: left colectomy with reanastomosis of transverse colon
>   Distal sigmoid and rectum: abdominal-perineal resection with permanent colostomy
- Discuss planned surgery with client; include content related to colostomy, appearance, and location of stoma.
- Preoperatively and postoperatively evaluate physical ability to do ostomy care (e.g., use of hands and fingers, eyesight, physical strength, willingness to learn); assist as necessary.
- Encourage client to express fears, grief, and anxiety concerning diagnosis and treatment.

- Allow client to regain physical and emotional strength before beginning postoperative teaching regarding ostomy care and diet.
- Teach client to observe for and report complications:
    Pain, redness, swelling
    Excoriated peristomal skin of incision
    Obstruction of output
    Stoma prolapse or retraction
    Altered stool consistency
- Provide client with written instructions concerning the following:
    Dietary considerations about foods that cause flatus (cabbage, beans, carbonated beverages) and blockage (nuts, spinach, lettuce, popcorn)
    Ostomy appliances: how to measure for size, where to buy
    Community resources (e.g., ostomy clubs)
- Refer to ostomy specialist as needed.

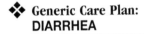 Generic Care Plan:
   DIARRHEA

GENERAL INFORMATION

Diarrhea is an increase in the amount and frequency of bowel movements. When diarrhea results from an infection, stools are watery and loose. Sometimes the rapid expulsion of stools causes a lack of bowel control or fecal incontinence, which improves when the diarrhea ceases.

CAUSATIVE/CONTRIBUTING FACTORS

Bacterial, viral, or parasitic infection
Drug reaction (e.g., antibiotics, laxatives)
Enzyme deficiency
Food allergy
Stress
Diverticulosis
Cancer
Nutritional supplements and enteral feedings
Malabsorption, vitamin deficiency

CLINICAL MANIFESTATIONS

Increased frequency and volume of stool
Watery stool
Abdominal cramping, pain
Nausea, vomiting
Malaise, possible fever
Dehydration
Perianal excoriation; burning sensation
Positive stool, blood culture
Delirium

NURSING PROCESS

Assessment Considerations

- History of frequent, watery stools
- Symptoms of electrolyte imbalance (see Table 5-5)
- History of possible causative factors (e.g., recent travel, drug regimen)
- Important to rule out fecal impaction, which can present with diarrhea-like signs

Goals

- Client reduces bowel movements to no more than one per day.
- Client reestablishes normal pattern of bowel elimination.
- Client has underlying cause of diarrhea treated.
- Client is free from dehydration, weakness, anal excoriation.

Nursing Interventions

- Assist with identifying and treating underlying cause.
- Record intake and output, number and character of stools, daily weight.
- Consider diarrhea a sign of infection until cause is determined; follow enteric precautions and monitor vital signs.
- Practice proper hand-washing technique before and after contact with client.
- Instruct client to cleanse and dry rectal area, apply petroleum gel to prevent excoriation; assist as needed.
- Observe for signs of dehydration (e.g., poor skin turgor, postural hypotension, sunken eyes, rapid pulse); increase intake of fluids, as tolerated, avoiding milk products.

- Administer intravenous fluids and electrolytes as ordered.
- Administer antidiarrheal agents as ordered; observe for change in stools, color, amount, and consistency.
- Teach client safe practices to avoid or control diarrhea (e.g., dietary practices, safe laxative use).

Evaluation
- Client exhibits normal elimination pattern.
- Client maintains normal perirectal skin integrity.
- Client possesses fluid and electrolyte balance.

Possible Related Nursing Diagnoses
Bowel incontinence
Fluid volume deficit
High risk for infection
Impaired skin integrity

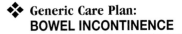

❖ Generic Care Plan:
BOWEL INCONTINENCE

GENERAL INFORMATION

Bowel incontinence refers to the inability to control the elimination of feces because of physical or cognitive disorders. Chronic fecal incontinence, which can appear as diarrhea, is usually associated with a neurologic deficit or disease of the colon, rectum, or anus.

CAUSATIVE/CONTRIBUTING FACTORS

Fecal impaction
Severe diarrhea
Carcinoma of the rectum
Prolapsed rectum
Debilitation and weakness causing the inability to exert muscular effort against a normal gastrocolic reflex
Inability to toilet independently
Cognitive deficit

CLINICAL MANIFESTATIONS

Uncontrolled passage of fecal matter

Neurogenic incontinence: incontinence once or twice per day

NURSING PROCESS

Assessment Considerations

- Frequency, characteristics, and amount of stool
- Precipitating factors
- Presence of neurologic or other disease
- Awareness of sensations signaling the need to defecate

BOX 6-1   Bowel Retraining

PURPOSE

To reestablish partial to full control of bowel movements

ASSESSMENT

Client's general physical and mental condition

Bowel and sphincter function

Cause, length of time, and degree of incontinence

Anticipated cooperation of client and family

PRELIMINARY ACTIONS

Keep record of client's bowel movement pattern: time, amount of stool, relationship to meals and activities.

Identify stimuli for bowel movement.

Identify client's ability to perceive need to have bowel movement.

PROCEDURE

Based on assessments, establish regular time when bowel movement can be anticipated and plan toileting at that time.

Insert a glycerin suppository into rectum approximately 30 minutes before scheduled time.

Position client in sitting position on bedpan or commode, out of bed if possible.

Place footstool under feet to promote bowel elimination.

Instruct client to take several deep breaths, tighten abdomen, press hands on abdomen to apply pressure and bear down; bending down also helps if client can tolerate it.

If there is no bowel movement after 10 minutes take patient off bedpan or commode.

Maintain a record of attempts and outcomes.

After a routine is established, mechanical stimulation through the use of a suppository may not be necessary.

- Mental status
- Self-care capacity

Goals
- The client regains bowel control and maintains regular pattern of bowel elimination.
- The client is free from skin breakdown.

Nursing Interventions
- Assist with identification and treatment of underlying cause.
- Record frequency, amount, and client's control of bowel movements.
- Ensure proper hygienic practices and thorough skin cleaning after bowel movements; keep skin clean and dry.
- Establish appropriate bowel retraining program (Box 6-1).

Evaluation
- Client establishes control of bowel movements.
- Client possesses intact skin around rectal area and buttocks.

Possible Related Nursing Diagnoses
Altered thought processes
Constipation
Diarrhea
High risk for fluid volume deficit
High risk for infection
Impaired skin integrity
Self-care deficit: toileting

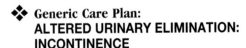

❖ Generic Care Plan:
ALTERED URINARY ELIMINATION: INCONTINENCE

GENERAL INFORMATION

Urinary incontinence is the inability to control the release of urine. There are various types of urinary incontinence:

> *Stress:* Weakness of supporting pelvic muscles that causes urine to be released through the bladder outlet when one coughs, laughs, sneezes, or exercises

Urge: Spasm or irritated bladder walls that cause sudden need to void and involuntary passage of urine

Reflex: Lack of sensation of signal to void leading to involuntary loss of urine when a specific volume of urine fills bladder

Overflow: Excess accumulation of urine in bladder because of failure of bladder muscles to contract or lack of relaxation of periurethral muscles

Total: Constant loss of urine without any appreciable volume accumulating in the bladder and without sensation

Functional: Existence of factor that interferes with the ability to toilet and that is unrelated to disorders of the urinary tract

Although not a normal outcome of aging, incontinence is more prevalent among older persons.

CAUSATIVE/CONTRIBUTING FACTORS

Pelvic muscle weakness or relaxation secondary to multiple pregnancies; reduction in estrogen; obesity

Urinary tract infection

Dehydration (concentrated urine irritates bladder wall)

Compression of urethra and bladder by prostatic hypertrophy, fecal impaction

Bladder neck obstruction

Neurologic disease (e.g., CVA, multiple sclerosis, Parkinson's disease)

Impaired cognition, depression

Confinement to bed

Inaccessible bathroom

Dependency on others for toileting

Medications (e.g., anticholinergics, adrenergic antagonists, diuretics)

CLINICAL MANIFESTATIONS

Involuntary loss of urine indicated by the following:
        Urine on floor
        Wet clothing, linens
        Urine odor
        Damp or stained clothing, furniture, floor
Frequent toileting, reluctance to be far from bathroom

NURSING PROCESS
Assessment Considerations
- Obtaining history regarding the following:
    Date of onset
    Pattern (e.g., constant dribbling, sudden expulsion of large amounts)
    Frequency and occurrence (during night, only when sneezing)
    Precipitating factors (e.g., delay in voiding, laughing, diuretics)
    Related factors (weight gain, constipation, new medication)
    Intake and output
    Client's reaction (e.g., unaware, embarrassed, socially isolated)
- Review of medications being taken for possible relationship
- Evaluation of functional status
- Inquiry about presence of other symptoms (e.g., abdominal pain, fever)
- Evaluation of neurologic and mental status
- Diagnostic tests
    Urinalysis
    Intravenous pyelogram (to determine renal function)
    Cystoscopy
    Cystometrogram (to determine pattern of bladder emptying)
    Cystometry (to determine motor and sensory function of bladder)

Goals
- Client regains bladder continence.
- Client maintains or regains positive self-concept and dignity.
- Client is free from secondary problems such as skin breakdown, social isolation, and falls.

Nursing Interventions
- Assist with identification and treatment of underlying cause; prepare client for diagnostic tests as necessary.
- Record and monitor intake and output; estimate and record urine output when client voids on clothing or linens (1 inch diameter = approximately 10 ml of urine).
- Provide easily accessible toilet facilities; arrange for bedside commode, if necessary; move client closer to bathroom.

- Reinforce appropriate toileting behavior by reminding the client to toilet frequently and avoid prolonged periods between toileting to prevent retention.
- Implement *prompted voiding procedure:*
  Check client for wetness.
  Periodically ask the client if he/she is wet or dry.
  Determine frequency and anticipated times for voiding.
  Instruct client to toilet at interval before anticipated time for voiding.
  Praise client for successfully toileting.

BOX 6-2 Bladder Retraining

PURPOSE
To reestablish partial to complete control of urinary elimination without urinary retention, overflow, or infection

ASSESSMENT
General physical and mental status
Urinary tract function; ability to regain continence
Cause, duration, and degree of incontinence
Anticipated cooperation of client and care givers

ACTIONS
- Encourage good fluid intake during the day (at least 1500 ml unless contraindicated); reduce but do not eliminate fluid intake after 8 PM.
- If diuretics are prescribed, administer early in the day.
- Periodically ask client if he/she is wet or dry; monitor interval between voiding.
- Record client's voiding pattern: time, amount voided, fluid intake, and related factors.
- Determine average time client can hold urine.
- Establish schedule of expected voiding times based on client's pattern.
- Toilet client approximately 30 minutes before expected voiding time.
- Encourage voiding by measures such as running water; instructing client to tighten and relax pelvic muscles or rock back and forth; or pouring a small amount of warm water over the vulva or penis.
- Measure the initial amount voided; then press the lower abdomen over the bladder to assist in expressing remaining urine (Credé's method); measure this amount.
- Praise client for appropriate toileting.
- If incontinent episode occurs, discuss with client to determine possible cause.
- Record results.

- Institute bladder retraining program if appropriate (Box 6-2).
- Provide devices to protect clothing and bedclothes such as urinary sheaths, condom catheters, adult briefs, and incontinence pants (unless bladder retraining program in effect).
- Avoid indwelling catheter use if possible; consult with physician regarding intermittent catheterization.
- Ensure client is cleansed with soap and water after incontinence (even if urine has dried, remaining crystals can cause irritation).
- Prevent accidents and injuries associated with incontinence:
    Provide good lighting to and inside bathroom.
    Answer calls for assistance promptly to prevent client from trying to climb over bed rails or attempting to independently ambulate inappropriately.
    Clean urine spills immediately.
- Modify environment to accommodate incontinence:
    Remove rugs so that floor can be cleaned when soiled.
    Use furniture with washable surfaces.
    Use a mattress with a washable surface or protect mattress with washable pads or covers.
    Provide good ventilation.
    Use room deodorizers as needed.
- Teach pelvic muscle exercises to females if good sensation and voluntary control over urine flow exist (helpful in controlling stress incontinence):
    Have client tighten anal sphincter for about 10 seconds as though holding in a bowel movement, then relax, tighten vagina as though stopping urinary flow, then relax.
    Repeat procedure several times each hour.
    Counsel client that exercises must be done regularly and consistently over several months to achieve results.
- Treat incontinent episodes in a matter-of-fact manner; do not chastise client or overemphasize the problem; discuss episode with client to help determine cause; reinforce teaching on prevention.
- Ensure client always has toileting facilities easily accessible.
- Encourage client to verbalize fears and concerns; encourage socialization and a normal life-style.
- Encourage client to limit oral intake after dinner and to reduce/eliminate intake of alcohol and caffeine-containing drinks.
- Teach self-catheterization, if indicated, and provide client with appropriate equipment; arrange for home health nursing referral as needed.

Evaluation
- Client is dry and odor free.
- Client uses toilet for voiding.
- Client is continent of urine.
- Client is free from complications secondary to incontinence.

Possible Related Nursing Diagnoses
High risk for infection
High risk for injury
High risk for impaired skin integrity
Self-care deficit: toileting
Social isolation

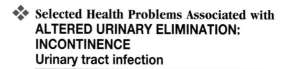

❖ **Selected Health Problems Associated with
ALTERED URINARY ELIMINATION:
INCONTINENCE
Urinary tract infection**

_____

GENERAL INFORMATION

A urinary tract infection is a bacterial invasion of the bladder or kidney. This is the most common infection in the elderly. The most common causes of urinary tract infection are *Escherichia coli* in women and *Proteus bacilli* in men.

CAUSATIVE/CONTRIBUTING FACTORS

Obstructions of urinary flow; calculi
Diabetes mellitus
Neurologic disorders that promote postvoiding residual urine
Atrophic vaginal mucosa; senile vaginitis
Frequent catheterizations
Indwelling catheters
Poor hygiene or wiping techniques in women
Immunologic disease

CLINICAL MANIFESTATIONS

Frequency, urgency
Burning in urethra

Bladder, kidney, or suprapubic pain
Elevated temperature
Blood and/or pus in urine
Urinary incontinence
Confusion

ADDITIONAL NURSING INTERVENTIONS
TO INCORPORATE INTO GENERIC CARE PLAN

- Assist with identification and treatment of underlying cause.
- Encourage fluids (about 2000 ml daily unless contraindicated).
- Observe quality of urine (e.g., color, odor) and pattern and frequency of urinary elimination; monitor intake and output.
- Prevent immobility and other sources of urinary stasis.
- Instruct client in proper wiping and hygienic practices, if necessary.
- Use adult briefs and other alternatives to indwelling catheters if incontinence is a problem; the risk of urinary tract infection increases significantly in catheterized persons.
- Use proper techniques to care for indwelling catheters (Box 6-3).

BOX 6-3 Indwelling Catheter Care

- Ensure indwelling catheters are used only when absolutely necessary for the clinical benefit of the client.
- Adhere to strict aseptic technique during catheterization.
- Secure the catheter so that it is not pulled or dislodged.
- Keep the drainage system closed.
- Prevent urine from backflowing in the catheter; ensure collection unit is positioned below level of client's bladder.
- Avoid and check for kinks in the tubing.
- Ensure client is not sitting on tubing and that obstructions to drainage flow are not present.
- Do not irrigate the catheter unless obstruction is present.
- If a urine specimen must be obtained, withdraw from the system with a sterile needle; adhere to aseptic technique.
- Maintain regular and meticulous cleanliness of perineal area, meatus, and drainage system.
- Observe for and promptly report signs of urinary tract infection (e.g., cloudy urine, elevated temperature, altered mental status, hematuria).

Benign prostatic hypertrophy

GENERAL INFORMATION

Enlargement of the prostate gland is common in late life and affects most elderly men. This enlargement can lead to bladder outlet obstruction, urinary retention, and a distended bladder.

CAUSATIVE/CONTRIBUTING FACTORS

Urinary frequency
Hesitancy
Dribbling
Nocturia
Weak flow (forked stream)
Recurrent urinary tract infections
Hematuria
In late stages there can be:
> Urinary retention
> Anorexia
> Incontinence
> Nausea, vomiting
> Weight loss, apathy

ADDITIONAL NURSING INTERVENTIONS
TO INCORPORATE INTO GENERIC CARE PLAN

- Assist with diagnosis and treatment of underlying cause; treatment can include the following:
  > Urinary antiseptics, if infection is present
  > Prostatic massage to relieve congestion
  > Medication to reduce benign prostatic hyperplasia
  > Surgical intervention (transurethral resection, open prostatectomy)
- Encourage good fluid intake during the day with reduced fluid intake at night.
- Monitor intake and output.
- Teach client about condition:
  > Most older men experience some degree of prostatic hypertrophy, most of which is benign.
  > Medical evaluation every 6 months is important in detecting

complications early; PSA (prostate-specific antigen) testing is advisable.

Clarify misconceptions concerning relationship of prostate problems to sexual function.

Reassure client that most prostate surgeries do not result in impotency to ensure that client will not be reluctant to have surgery for this reason.

RECOMMENDED READINGS

Brink CA, Sampselle CM, Wells TJ et al: A digital test for pelvic muscle strength in older women with urinary incontinence, *Nurs Res* 38:196, 1989.

Cunha BA, Marx J, Gingrich D: Managing prostatitis in the elderly, *Geriatrics* 46(1):60, 1991.

Loughlin KR: Medical and nonmedical therapies for benign prostatic hypertrophy, *Geriatrics* 46(6):26, 1991.

National Institutes of Health Consensus Development Conference: Urinary incontinence in adults, *J Am Geriatr Soc* 38(3):265, 1990.

Palmer MH, McCormick KA: Alterations in elimination: urinary incontinence. In Baines EM editor: *Perspectives on gerontological nursing,* Newbury Park, CA, 1991, Sage.

Wells TJ: Conquering incontinence, *Geriatr Nurs* 11(3):133, 1990.

7

❖ Activity and Exercise

G rowing numbers of Americans are aware of the benefits of exercise, contributing to increasing numbers of persons aging in more active states than previously. An active state is highly beneficial to older adults. Activity promotes lung expansion, circulation, digestion, elimination, muscle tone, bone strength, and other aspects of physical health. Healthy mental and social functioning is promoted, and, in addition, many of the elderly's health risks can be minimized by activity.

As advantageous as it is, activity is not necessarily an easy task for many older adults. Stiff joints, shortness of breath, weak muscles, poor coordination, fatigue, and other disorders can make movement difficult. Other factors that restrict older adults' social activity can be a limited budget or not having access to transportation. Inactivity can easily result from the common problems and changes the elderly face. Once inactive, the elderly are at risk for serious threats to their physical, mental, and social well-being, compounding other preexisting problems.

Activity depends on many physical and psychosocial factors, including well-functioning respiratory and cardiac systems; adequate nutrition; the ability to be mobile; pain-free joints; normal cognition and mood; good energy level; and the desire to participate in work and leisure. Age-related changes, disability, and illness can impact these factors and impair activity in a variety of ways.

Gerontologic nurses should assess potential and actual risks to activity and use a wide range of interventions to promote the maximum level of activity within the limitations of age and illness.

❖ Generic Care Plan:
INEFFECTIVE AIRWAY CLEARANCE

GENERAL INFORMATION

Ineffective airway clearance is an impairment to the passage of air through the respiratory tract because of the presence of an obstruction or because of the inability to effectively clear secretions.

CAUSATIVE/CONTRIBUTING FACTORS

Age-related changes to respiratory system
Obstruction or infection of the trachea and/or bronchi
Excess bronchial secretions
Fatigue, decreased mobility
Trauma
Cognitive/perceptual impairment

CLINICAL MANIFESTATIONS

Abnormal breath sounds: crackles (rales), rhonchi
Changes in rate and depth of respirations
Tachypnea
Dyspnea, cyanosis
Cough: older adults have less effective cough response
Fever
        May be atypical
        Respiratory infections are second most common cause of
            temperature elevation in the elderly
Altered mental status

NURSING PROCESS

Assessment Considerations
- Breath sounds; rate and depth of respirations
- Client's color: skin, nail beds, mucous membranes
- Vital signs
- Presence and characteristics of cough
- Sputum characteristics
- Posture
- Activity level

- Level of comfort
- Appetite; nutritional status
- Smoking and allergy history
- Status of pneumococcal and influenza vaccinations

Goals
- Client maintains or regains patent airway, optimal respirations.
- Client effectively expectorates secretions from airway.
- Client is free from infection.

Nursing Interventions
- Prepare client for diagnostic procedures, as necessary:
    Chest x-ray film
    Pulmonary function test
    Sputum cultures and cytology
- Assist with prescribed treatments:
    Intermittent positive-pressure breathing (IPPB)
    Oxygen therapy
    Suctioning
    Postural drainage
    Medications: antibiotics, steroids, cough preparations, bronchodilators, antipyretics
- Encourage deep breathing, coughing every 2 hours.
- Ensure fluid intake of at least 1500 ml (unless contraindicated) to liquefy secretions; offer fluids hourly.
- Humidify breathed air (use humidifier or place pan containing water on top of radiator or other heat source).
- Provide foods that are easily chewed and swallowed if client is severely dyspneic.
- Offer frequent oral hygiene to increase comfort and promote appetite.
- Monitor vital signs, breath sounds, sputum production, color, and level of consciousness at least every 4 hours.
- Monitor effects of medications, client's comfort.
- Provide and encourage use of tissues for disposal of expectorated matter.
- Ensure client takes or receives prescribed antibiotics on time and that the entire prescription is consumed; assess for related complications.
- Teach client early signs of respiratory infection (e.g., increased cough; increased production and/or viscosity of sputum; change in sputum color to yellow, green, or gray; tightness in chest; dyspnea; fever).

- Teach client and care givers prevention measures:
    Avoidance of contact with persons with respiratory illness
    Breathing exercises, good breathing techniques
    Regular activity
    Avoidance of cigarette smoke
    Good nutrition
    Annual influenza vaccine; one-time pneumococcal vaccine

Evaluation
- Client breathes at a rate and depth within a normal range.
- Client's sputum production decreases.
- Client's vital signs are within normal range.
- Client has normal color.
- Client is free from abnormal breath sounds, dyspnea, shortness of breath.
- Client receives annual influenza vaccine.

Possible Related Nursing Diagnoses
Altered nutrition: less than body requirements
Altered thought processes
Anxiety
Fatigue
High risk for infection
Impaired gas exchange
Sleep pattern disturbance

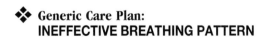

❖ Generic Care Plan:
INEFFECTIVE BREATHING PATTERN

GENERAL INFORMATION

Ineffective breathing pattern exists when inhalation or expiration patterns prevent adequate ventilation to meet individual pulmonary needs.

CAUSATIVE/CONTRIBUTING FACTORS

Age-related changes to respiratory system
Decreased energy, fatigue
Immobility
Pain, especially postoperative

Decreased lung expansion
Tracheobronchial obstruction
Neuromuscular or musculoskeletal impairment

CLINICAL MANIFESTATIONS

Dyspnea, shortness of breath
Tachypnea
Fremitus
Cyanosis
Cough
Nasal flaring
Changes in respiratory depth
Pursed-lip breathing, prolonged expiratory phase
Increased anteroposterior diameter
Use of accessory muscles
Altered chest excursion

NURSING PROCESS

Assessment Considerations

- Type of breathing pattern (e.g., tachypnea, Cheyne-Stokes)
- Breath sounds
- Pain, discomfort
- Emotional response
- Results of laboratory studies, arterial blood gases

Goals

- Client demonstrates appropriate breathing techniques.
- Client possesses normal arterial blood gases.

Nursing Interventions

- Prepare client for diagnostic tests, such as arterial blood gases.
- Assist with prescribed treatments as necessary:
    IPPB
    Oxygen therapy
    Bronchodilators
- Ask client to take five deep breaths and evaluate quality of respirations: short breaths and movement of the shoulders indicate shallow breathing; contraction of the abdomen during inspiration indicates poor use of diaphragm. Teach proper mechanics for breathing:

The abdomen, not the chest, should move: during inspiration abdomen should protrude and sink; during expiration abdomen should pull in and upward.

Have the client monitor movement by placing one hand on the abdomen and one on the chest; only the hand on the abdomen should move during respiration (Figure 7-1).

- Teach a rate of breathing that facilitates good air exchange:

Focus on forcing air out of the lungs (age-related changes can result in less elastic recoil of lungs and lead to some carbon dioxide remaining in lungs).

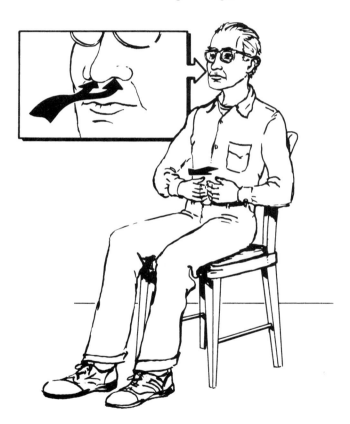

FIGURE 7-1 Clients can be taught exercises to strengthen the diaphragm muscle. Inhaling air should cause hands to move out with expanding of the abdomen. During exhalation, abdomen and hands will move in again. (From Hoeman S: *Rehabilitation/restorative care in the community,* St Louis, 1990, Mosby–Year Book.)

Instruct client to inhale to the count of 1 and exhale for 3 counts.

Have client repeat exercises several times throughout the day; five repetitions of each exercise at each session are sufficient initially but gradually increase this number.

Inform client that in addition to promoting respiratory activity, breathing exercises also help to relieve stress and promote relaxation.

- Conserve client's energy and promote good nutritional status by providing small meals at frequent intervals.
- Administer analgesics as ordered.
- Monitor vital signs, respiratory rate and depth.

Evaluation
- Client is free from nasal flaring, use of accessory respiratory muscles.
- Client performs breathing exercises at least three times daily.

Possible Related Nursing Diagnoses
Activity intolerance
Altered nutrition: less than body requirements
Altered thought processes
Altered tissue perfusion
Anxiety
Fatigue
High risk for infection
Impaired gas exchange

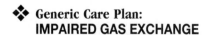

❖ Generic Care Plan:
IMPAIRED GAS EXCHANGE

GENERAL INFORMATION

Impaired gas exchange occurs when there is a decreased passage of gases (O_2, CO_2) between the alveoli of the lungs and the vascular system. In addition to hypoxia, excessive oxygen administration has serious implications for the older adult. High levels of oxygen can depress the respiratory center and interfere with carbon dioxide elimination. Carbon dioxide retention results, leading to potentially fatal acidosis and carbon dioxide narcosis.

CAUSATIVE/CONTRIBUTING FACTORS

Age-related changes to respiratory system
Altered oxygen supply
Alveolocapillary membrane changes
Altered blood flow
Altered oxygen-carrying capacity of blood

CLINICAL MANIFESTATIONS

Skin color changes, cyanosis
Respiratory changes: increased respirations (also may be shallow and slow), air hunger, dyspnea, shortness of breath
Altered mental status: confusion, anxiety, irritability, restlessness, altered level of consciousness
Drowsiness, fatigue
Poor coordination, slurred speech, slowed reaction time
Anorexia, weight loss
Physical signs (late chronic signs): clubbing, barrel chest
Abnormal arterial blood gases, depressed PO_2, increased PCO_2 (compensatory acidosis)

NURSING PROCESS

Assessment Considerations

- Respirations and breath sounds
- Skin color
- Mental status and level of consciousness
- Posture and coordination
- Energy level
- Appetite
- Blood gases

Goals

- Client possesses arterial blood gases within normal range.
- Client is free from complications related to oxygen therapy.

Nursing Interventions

- Prepare client for diagnostic tests, such as pulmonary function and arterial blood gases.
- Administer bronchodilators or expectorants as prescribed: Evaluate effects.

- Use the most effective method of oxygen administration:
    Avoid use of nasal cannula if client breathes through the mouth.
    Avoid face mask if client is emaciated.
    Maintain level of oxygen administration between 2 and 3 L/min unless otherwise instructed.
    Check client and equipment at least hourly.
    Check blood gas results frequently.
- Monitor for signs of CO_2 narcosis (decreased respirations, headache, flushing, altered level of consciousness, increased PO_2, and increased PCO_2).
- Provide proper care for nasal cannulas.
    Keep humidifier filled with distilled water.
    Ensure that the prongs stay in the nostrils.
    Place gauze between tubing and skin surface over the ears; observe for signs of skin irritation and breakdown.
    Lubricate lips and nose with water-soluble (not petroleum-based) lubricant jelly.
    Provide regular oral and nasal hygiene.
- Closely monitor client's vital signs, mental status, and skin color.
- Post *Oxygen In Use, NO SMOKING* signs and enforce them.
- Check oxygen equipment and setting at least hourly.
- Avoid use of alcohol or petroleum-based products in care.
- Protect client from static electricity and hazardous electrical appliances.
- Promote good fluid intake.
- Encourage client to frequently turn, cough, and deep breathe.
- Raise head of bed 30 degrees unless contraindicated.
- Encourage activity as tolerated.
- Have frequent contact with client.

Evaluation
- Client has PO_2 above 60 mm Hg and PCO_2 between 35 and 45 mm Hg.
- Client demonstrates normal cognition and level of consciousness.
- Client has good skin color.
- Client breathes comfortably.
- Client is free from complications related to oxygen therapy.

Possible Related Nursing Diagnoses
Activity intolerance
Altered thought processes
Anxiety
Fatigue
High risk for injury
Ineffective airway clearance
Sleep pattern disturbance

 **Selected Health Problems Associated with
IMPAIRED GAS EXCHANGE:
Pneumonia**

GENERAL INFORMATION

Pneumonia ranks with influenza as the fourth leading cause of death in older adults. The elderly are at particularly high risk because of their reduced respiratory activity, decreased ability to effectively remove secretions, decreased resistance, and presence of other conditions that reduce activity. The effects of this inflammation of the lung can be devastating. The most common form of pneumonia in community-based elderly is pneumococcal pneumonia; *Klebsiella, Pseudomonas aeruginosa, Enterobacter, Escherichia coli,* and other gram-negative bacilli are more common in institutionalized elderly. The pattern of onset varies. Pneumococcal and *Klebsiella* pneumonias have a rapid onset with shaking and chills; stapylococcal pneumonias develop slowly and subtly.

CAUSATIVE/CONTRIBUTING FACTORS

Age-related changes to respiratory system
Aspiration
Upper respiratory infections (especially influenza)
Impaired respirations as a result of debilitation, immobility
Chronic obstructive pulmonary disease
Increased bronchial secretion
Postoperative weakness

CLINICAL MANIFESTATIONS

Altered mental status
Temperature elevation
Elevated pulse
Rapid respiration
Productive cough; pink to rust-colored mucus
Cyanosis
Crackles (rales)
Anorexia, weight loss
Consolidation (visible on chest x-ray film)
Elevated white blood cell count (WBC)

ADDITIONAL NURSING INTERVENTIONS TO INCORPORATE INTO GENERIC CARE PLAN

- Assist with diagnostic tests, such as x-ray film and sputum and blood cultures.
- Administer antibiotics (see Box 4-1), analgesics (see Table 8-1), antipyretics, and cough preparations as prescribed; monitor effects. Ensure antibiotic doses are given completely and on time to maintain appropriate blood levels.
- Monitor oxygen therapy.
- Observe closely for signs of complications (septicemia, paralytic ileus, atelectasis, lung abscess, congestive heart failure, dysrhythmias, delirium, meningitis).
- Provide comfort measures, such as offering fluids, raising head of bed, changing damp bed linens, repositioning.
- If intravenous lines are used, monitor closely.

Emphysema

GENERAL INFORMATION

Chronic obstructive pulmonary disease (COPD) is a destructive lung condition that can include a variety of diseases that obstruct airflow. Emphysema is an example of COPD and is characterized by a distension and reduction in number of alveoli. Emphysema is a common finding among older adults, with a higher prevalence among cigarette smokers. The progression of emphysema is gradual.

CAUSATIVE/CONTRIBUTING FACTORS

Cigarette smoking

Heredity (inherited deficiency in protein alpha$_1$ antitrypsin that leads to destruction of lung tissue)

Age-related changes to respiratory system

Allergy

Chronic bronchitis with repeated infection

Chronic irritation, such as air pollution, occupational contact

CLINICAL MANIFESTATIONS

Slow, subtle onset of symptoms

Ruddy, pink complexion from hypoxia caused by high blood CO_2 level

Expiratory difficulties

Dyspnea, shortness of breath, wheezing, pursed-lip breathing

Tendency to prefer sitting position with elbows on thighs for ease in breathing

Chronic cough with sputum production

Weakness, lethargy

Anorexia, weight loss

ADDITIONAL NURSING INTERVENTIONS
TO INCORPORATE INTO GENERIC CARE PLAN

- Assist with postural drainage and IPPB as necessary.
- Keep oxygen administration ≤2 L/min to avoid complications. Instruct client and care givers in safe use of home oxygen (Box 7-1).
- Determine impact of disease on functional ability:
    Ask about ability to participate in activities of daily living.
    Review effects of disease on appetite, sleep, energy, cognition, and other functional aspects.
    Explore client's and family's emotional reaction to the disease; provide counseling and support.
- Teach realities and care of disease (e.g., prophylactic use of antibiotics, breathing exercises, recognition of complications).
- Instruct in identifying and avoiding environmental factors that can worsen condition (e.g., high humidity, pollution, extremes in temperature, cigarette smoke).
- If client smokes, assist with smoking cessation efforts.

BOX 7-1   Guidelines for Safe Use of Home Oxygen

- Remove fire hazards from environment.
- Instruct all persons in the home that smoking is not allowed; post no smoking signs.
- Teach family proper use of oxygen, including signs of complications.
- Secure the oxygen tank in a stand, in a safe location, at least 6 feet away from heat sources and electrical appliances.
- Keep oil, grease, alcohol, and other combustibles away from the area in which oxygen is used.
- Have a fire extinguisher readily available.
- Notify the local fire department that oxygen is in use at the client's address.
- Close valves of tank when not in use.
- Post the prescribed setting on tank and reinforce the importance of not changing the setting.

Chronic bronchitis

GENERAL INFORMATION

Chronic bronchitis is another form of COPD, characterized by a chronic inflammation of the bronchi with production of a large amount of sputum that results in bronchial obstruction. Symptoms develop gradually, often over years, and are most prevalent during cold weather.

CAUSATIVE/CONTRIBUTING FACTORS

Infections of the respiratory tract (pneumonia, acute bronchitis)
Irritation of the bronchial tree (e.g., dusts, smoking)
Heredity

CLINICAL MANIFESTATIONS

Recurrent productive cough
Frequent acute respiratory infections followed by lingering cough
Production of thick sputum
Dyspnea or shortness of breath
Wheezing

ADDITIONAL NURSING INTERVENTIONS
TO INCORPORATE INTO GENERIC CARE PLAN

- Identify and remove irritants in the environment (e.g., dust, pets).
- Assist client in smoking cessation efforts.
- Limit client's exposure to cigarette smoke and other pollutants.
- Explore occupational factors that could contribute to respiratory problems.
- Administer or instruct client to administer antibiotics, bronchodilators, steroids, and other medications, as prescribed.
- Assist with IPPB treatments as ordered.

Tuberculosis (TB)

GENERAL INFORMATION

Tuberculosis is a disease that most commonly affects the lungs and is caused by *Mycobacterium tuberculosis*. Most cases of TB in older adults are reactivations of earlier infections. The elderly are at increased risk of developing TB from direct exposure because of poor resistance to infections and the high prevalence of chronic diseases or debilitating conditions.

CAUSATIVE/CONTRIBUTING FACTORS

Infection with tuberculosis bacillus; reactivation of earlier infection
Residing in high-density area
Debilitated state

CLINICAL MANIFESTATIONS

Fatigue
Anorexia, weight loss, cachexia
Productive cough (often blood tinged)
Temperature elevation (usually low grade)
Night sweats may not occur because of decreased diaphoresis in late life

ADDITIONAL NURSING INTERVENTIONS
TO INCORPORATE INTO GENERIC CARE PLAN

- Recognize that a two-step Mantoux test is recommended in the elderly because of the high risk of false-negative results from a single test. If the initial test is negative, repeat in 1 week.
- Positive purified protein derivative (PPD) tests should be followed by chest x-ray film and clinical evaluation. TB in the elderly may present atypically on chest x-ray film.
- Administer medications as prescribed. Observe for adverse effects, particularly signs of hepatitis (e.g., jaundice, fever, anorexia, dark urine).
- Limit droplet spread by using tissues for secretions and instructing client to cover mouth when sneezing or coughing.
- Follow good hand-washing technique.
- Encourage good nutrition.
- Promote normal activities of daily living.
- Keep the environment clean and well ventilated.
- Arrange for diagnostic testing and follow-up care as needed.
- Screen elderly in institutional or group settings annually.

❖ **Generic Care Plan:**
ALTERED CARDIAC OUTPUT:
DECREASED

GENERAL INFORMATION

Decreased cardiac output exists when there is a reduction in the amount of blood pumped by the heart, resulting in inadequate circulation to the body's tissues.

CAUSATIVE/CONTRIBUTING FACTORS

Hypertension
Atherosclerosis
Conductive defects of heart
Congestive heart failure
Myocardial or valvular disease
Chronic obstructive pulmonary disease
Fluid and electrolyte imbalances

Shock, sepsis, allergic responses
Increased tissue demands for oxygen (e.g., fever, chronic anemia, malnutrition)
Age-related changes: reduced myocardial efficiency, weaker contractile force, more rigid valves, less elastic vessels, poor tolerance of tachycardia

CLINICAL MANIFESTATIONS

Fatigue
Dyspnea, crackles (rales), orthopnea, shortness of breath
Cough, frothy sputum
Decreased peripheral pulses, jugular vein distension
Dysrhythmias or electrocardiogram (ECG) changes
Cyanosis, pallor of skin
Cold, clammy skin
Edema
Oliguria
Delirium

NURSING PROCESS

Assessment Considerations
- Vital signs
- Quality of respirations, breath sounds
- Skin color, temperature, moisture
- Behavior (e.g., restlessness), cognition
- Level of consciousness
- Appetite, weight changes

Goals
- Client possesses normal heart rate and rhythm.
- Client is free from complications related to decreased cardiac output.

Nursing Interventions
- Monitor vital signs every 4 hours; if client is placed on cardiac monitor, observe cardiac rate and rhythm.
- Obtain baseline and regular reevaluations of ECG, electrolytes, serum creatinine, and blood urea nitrogen (BUN).
- Observe for and obtain prompt treatment for hypoxia.

- Monitor oxygen and intravenous therapy if ordered.
- Assist client in obtaining rest and comfort:
    Elevate head of bed to reduce pulmonary venous congestion.
    Encourage client to turn, cough, and deep breathe hourly.
    Implement passive exercises.
    Be alert to complications related to bed rest (e.g., pulmonary embolism, phlebothrombosis).
- Modify activity to prevent fatigue:
    Schedule rest periods after periods of activity.
    Provide nonstressful diversional activities.
    Encourage increase in activity as soon as allowed.
- Offer explanations, reassurance, and support to minimize anxiety.
- Monitor sleep and rest:
    Provide quiet, non-stimulating environment.
    Offer soft music if this aids client in relaxing.
    Schedule activities to maximize sleep periods.
    Consult with physician regarding use of sedatives if necessary.
- Administer and evaluate effects of diuretics (Table 7-1):
    Monitor intake and output; the elderly are highly susceptible to excessive diuresis when taking these drugs.
    Weigh daily.
    Review client's history for conditions that would contraindicate or warrant special caution with diuretic administration (e.g., anuria, hepatic or renal disease).
    Administer diuretics in the morning to minimize nocturia.
    Observe for signs of hypokalemia.
    Include high-potassium foods in diet to prevent toxicity (Box 7-2).
    Administer potassium supplements if prescribed.
- Administer and evaluate effects of antidysrhythmics (Table 7-2); be familiar with effects and contraindications (Table 7-3):
    Atropine: anticholinergic, blocks parasympathetic nerve impulses, can increase intraocular pressure when combined with haloperidol
    Lidocaine: treatment of choice in initial management of ventricular tachycardia, needs low infusion rate to avoid central nervous system (CNS) toxicity
    Phenytoin: similar action to procainamide and quinidine
    Procainamide: similar action to quinidine, better tolerated,

TABLE 7-1 Diuretics

Diuretics	Side effects	Nursing implications
Chlorothiazide (Diuril)	Headache, drowsiness, orthostatic hypotension, lethargy, confusion	Administer diuretics in morning to minimize nocturia
Hydrochlorothiazide (HydroDiuril)	Indigestion, nausea, vomiting, diarrhea	Do not restrict fluids without explicit medical justification
Spironolactone (Aldactone)	Photosensitivity	Prevent side effects by monitoring blood pressure, intake and output, vital signs, blood composition
Furosemide (Lasix)	Fluid/electrolyte imbalances Aplastic anemia, agranulocytosis, leukopenia, thrombocytopenia Reduced glucose tolerance Ringing in ears associated with furosemide toxicity Concurrent use of aminoglycoside antibiotics, some diuretics (ethacrynate sodium, furosemide) carry high risk of ototoxicity Simultaneous use of cortisone can cause excessive potassium depletion High risk of dysrhythmias when diuretics taken with digitalis preparations	Observe for specific concerns: • Hyponatremia (sodium below 125 mEq/L) • Low blood volume; reduced cardiac output Be alert to signs of dehydration: weakness, irritability, muscle cramps, fainting (may indicate fluid/electrolyte imbalance, which increases risk of digitalis toxicity and dysrhythmias) Encourage consumption of potassium-rich foods (see Box 7-2) Observe for subtle indications of infection and hyperglycemia (especially in diabetic patients)

Interactions: all diuretics
Increase effect of antihypertensives.
Decrease effect of allopurinol, digitalis preparations, oral anticoagulants, oral antidiabetic drugs, insulin, probenecid.
Effects increased by barbiturates, analgesics, any drug that can lower blood pressure.
Effects decreased by cholestryamine (do not take less than 1 hour before diuretic), large quantities of aspirin.

BOX 7-2   Potassium-Rich Foods

All-bran cereals	Milk
Almonds	Molasses
Apricots	Nectarines
Asparagus	Orange juice
Bananas	Oysters
Bass	Peaches
Beans (navy and lima)	Peanuts
Beef	Peanut butter
Brussel sprouts	Peas
Cabbage	Peppers
Carrots	Perch
Chicken	Plums
Citrus fruits	Pork
Coconut	Prunes
Crackers (graham and rye)	Raisins
Dates	Salmon
Figs	Sardines
Flounder	Scallops
Haddock	Spinach
Halibut	Sweet potatoes
Lamb	Tomatoes
Lentils	Tuna
Liver (beef)	Turkey

Consider sodium/calorie restrictions when including items in client's diet.

---

can cause muscle weakness and impaired breathing when taken with kanamycin, neomycin, or streptomycin
- Administer and monitor effects of medications:
    Ensure that initially smaller doses are administered until response is determined.
    Ensure serum levels of drugs are checked regularly; note possible toxic levels:
        Lidocaine: ≥ 5 µg/ml
        Phenytoin: ≥ 20 µg/ml
        Digoxin (Lanoxin): ≥ 2 ng/ml
        Procainamide: ≥ 8 µg/ml
        Quinidine: ≥ 8 µg/ml (quinidine has unpredictable effects, high risk of toxicity, prolonged time for elimination)

Text continued on p.164.

TABLE 7–2 Antidysrhythmics

General nursing measures

Remove potential hazards from environment (e.g., chemicals that could be
  accidentally ingested, clutter on floors).
Listen carefully to expressed needs and problems.
Advise client to change positions slowly and
  hold rails when climbing stairs.
Arrange for and monitor blood work.
Monitor nutritional status, intake and output, vital signs.

Drug	Side effects	Nursing implications
Atropine	Dry mouth, blurred vision, urinary retention, disorientation, constipation, tachycardia, heat stroke	Offer hard candies and good oral hygiene Keep oriented
Lidocaine	Confusion, slurred speech, depression, convulsions, bradycardia, tinnitus, blurred/double vision, dizziness	Keep airway tongue depressor in client's room
Phenytoin	Thrombocytopenia, leukopenia, ataxia, slurred speech, double/blurred vision, hyperglycemia	
Procainamide	Thrombocytopenia, hallucinations, confusion, bradycardia, anorexia, diarrhea, lupus erythematosus syndrome	Modify environment to avoid misperceptions Arrange for treatment of joint pain, muscle aches, fever, rash, and other symptoms related to lupus
Propranolol	Lethargy, cold extremities, bradycardia, reduced WBC, diarrhea, hypoglycemia	Protect from and observe for signs of infection Maintain body warmth; ensure client does not incur burns in effort to keep extremities warm (e.g., inappropriate use of hot water bottle or soaks)

Continued.

TABLE 7–2   Antidysrhythmics—cont'd

Drug	Side effects	Nursing implications
Quinidine	Serious dysrhythmia, hemolytic anemia, thrombocytopenia, vertigo, confusion, cold sweat, restlessness, tinnitus, excessive salivation, diarrhea, abdominal pain, asthma	Promote orientation Facilitate relaxation Keep dry; guard against skin breakdown

Interactions: all antidysrhythmics

Increase effect of insulin, oral antidiabetic drugs, anticoagulants, antihypertensives, atropine-like drugs, barbiturates.

Decrease effects of pilocarpine eye drops, cortisone, antihistamines, antiinflammatory drugs, myasthenia gravis drugs.

Effects increased by atropine-like drugs (e.g., antidepressants, antiparkinsonism drugs, antipsychotics), aspirin, coumarin preparations, estrogen, phenytoin.

Effects decreased by vitamin C, alcohol.

TABLE 7–3   Contraindications to Antidysrhythmic Use

Drug	Contraindications/cautions	Comments
Atropine	Open-angle glaucoma, chronic bronchitis, prostate enlargement, myasthenia gravis, peptic ulcer	Antidote: physostigmine salicylate
Lidocaine	Use with caution in all elderly; renal/hepatic diseases, congestive heart failure, weight below 100 lb	
Procainamide	Severe peripheral artery disease, bronchospasms, hypoglycemia (or tendency), congestive heart failure, respiratory disease	Antagonists: isoproterenol, glucagon
Quinidine	Myasthenia gravis, hyperthyroidism, recent use of digitalis, congestive heart failure, impaired myocardial function	

TABLE 7-4   Cardiac Glycosides

Drug	Side effects	Nursing implications
Digoxin (Lanoxin) Digitalis Digitoxin (Crystodigin) Lanatoside C (Cediland D) Quabain (G-strophanthin)	Confusion, memory loss, personality change, apathy, irritability, agitation, hallucinations, delirium, depression, impaired color vision, headache, fatigue, drowsiness, dizziness, aphasia, ataxia, fainting, seizures Muscle pain and weakness, neuralgias, restlessness, nightmares, insomnia, anorexia, nausea, vomiting Bradycardia, congestive heart failure, premature ventricular contraction, premature atrial contraction, paroxysmal atrial tachycardia, atrial fibrillation, ventricular tachycardia or fibrillation, SA block, premature AV nodal contraction High serum levels of drug 2 ng/ml digoxin 30 ng/ml digitoxin	Ensure smaller doses are utilized; half-life of cardiac glycosides is prolonged in elderly. Therapeutic doses must be individually calculated. Monitor digoxin blood level and observe for signs of digitalis toxicity (classic symptoms of anorexia, nausea, and vomiting do not occur as commonly among older persons; confusion and heart failure may be first clue). Be aware if client has hypothyroidism because this further decreases drug tolerance; hyperthyroid patients may require larger doses to achieve described effects. Review client's history for conditions contraindicating or requiring special caution in cardiac glycoside administration (e.g., anemia, rheumatic carditis, subacute bacterial endocarditis, hypocalcemia, antibiotic therapy). Review client's history for conditions that increase risk of toxicity (e.g., thyroid disease, severe cardiac disease, respiratory disease, reduced renal function, small body size, diuretic therapy, hypokalemia).

Continued.

TABLE 7-4   Cardiac Glycosides—cont'd

Drug	Side effects	Nursing implications
		Evaluate apical-radical pulse for 1 full minute before administration. Instruct client and caretaker in procedure.
		Assess for side effect of gynecomastia (enlargement and/or sensitivity of male breast tissue).
		Observe closely for signs of toxicity and monitor pulse closely. If toxicity develops, discontinue drug, notify physician, and monitor cardiac status.
		Review all drugs administered for potential interactions. Avoid concurrent use of adrenalin and cardiac glycosides because serious toxicity can result.

Interactions: all cardiac glycosides
Effects increased by guanethidine, phenytoin, propranolol, quinidine; any drug that reduces gastric motility.
Effects decreased by antacids, cholestyramine, kaolin-pectin, laxatives, neomycin, phenobarbital, phenylbutazone, rifampin.
Serious toxicity can result when cardiac glycosides are taken with cortisone, diuretics, parenteral calcium, reserpine, thyroid preparations.

Review other medications client is taking; consult with physician if client is taking other drugs with anticholinergic properties (e.g., antipsychotics, antidepressants, antiparkinsonism agents).
Administer and evaluate effects of cardiac glycosides (Table 7-4).
• Prevent alterations to skin integrity:
Change positions frequently.

Keep pressure off edematous extremities.
Keep linens dry and wrinkle free.
- Advise client as follows:
    Administer medications properly; instruct as needed.
    Monitor pulse.
    Wear ID bracelet indicating use of cardiac glycosides.
    Store medications in tightly closed containers, away from
        light.
    Follow dietary restrictions if indicated.
    Report symptoms to health care professions (e.g., sudden
        weight gain, chest pain, fatigue, dyspnea).

Evaluation
- Client has heart rate and rhythm within normal limits.
- Client is free from complications related to drug therapy.

Possible Related Nursing Diagnoses
Activity intolerance
Altered fluid volume: excess
Altered nutrition: less than body requirements
Anxiety
Fatigue
High risk for impaired skin integrity
Impaired gas exchange

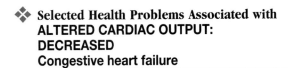

❖ Selected Health Problems Associated with ALTERED CARDIAC OUTPUT: DECREASED
Congestive heart failure

GENERAL INFORMATION

Congestive heart failure is a condition in which the heart is unable to pump an adequate amount of blood to meet the metabolic needs of the tissues. It increases in incidence with age and is a chronic condition for most people who experience this problem.

CAUSATIVE/CONTRIBUTING FACTORS

Congenital heart disease
Rheumatic heart disease
Hypertension

Mitral stenosis
Coronary heart disease
Corpulmonale
Acute myocardial infarction
Pulmonary emboli or infection
Ectopic rhythm
Fluid overload

CLINICAL MANIFESTATIONS

Shortness of breath
Fatigue
Anorexia or nausea
Unexplained and rapid weight gain
Dyspnea at rest (with advanced cardiac congestion)
Unbalanced fluid intake and output
Altered cognition, depression, or agitation
Insomnia or night wandering
Left-sided failure
    Dyspnea on exertion
    Orthopnea
    Paroxysmal nocturnal dyspnea
    Cough (early clue)
    Nocturia
    Crackles (rales), wheezes
Right-sided failure
    Distended neck veins
    Symmetric peripheral edema
    Hepatitic enlargement and tenderness
    Abdominal distension
    Ascites
    Gastrointestinal discomfort

ADDITIONAL NURSING INTERVENTIONS TO INCORPORATE INTO GENERIC CARE PLAN

- Review history of symptoms, onset, duration, and precipitating factors.
- Prepare client for diagnostic tests as indicated (e.g., x-ray, ECG, echocardiography).
- Support treatment plan (e.g., oxygen, diuretics [see Table 7-1], digitalis [see Table 7-4], vasodilators).
- Assess degree of pain, respiratory difficulty, nausea, fatigue,

presence of shock or impending shock, and skin color. Monitor vital signs, heart and breath sounds, fluid intake, and urinary output.
- Educate client about the physiologic changes that have occurred and the need to make life-style adjustments.
- Instruct client to weigh self daily to monitor weight loss or gain and possible fluid retention.
- Review client's understanding of medications; instruct as necessary.
- Teach client how to do leg exercises in bed to prevent phlebothrombosis.
- Monitor client's skin status; ensure client changes positions frequently. (Risk for skin breakdown is high.)
- Encourage frequent rest periods in presence of dyspnea, fatigue, or abnormal pulse rate.
- Instruct client to report symptoms such as swelling of ankles, feet, or abdomen; loss of appetite; weight gain; shortness of breath.

Myocardial infarction

GENERAL INFORMATION

Myocardial infarction is the lack of blood supply to the myocardium that results in tissue damage. Atypical signs and symptoms occur among the elderly; the first major clue can be confusion. Older adults tend to experience larger infarctions and a higher incidence of mortality, heart failure, pulmonary edema, and ventricular rupture.

CAUSATIVE/CONTRIBUTING FACTORS

Atherosclerotic heart disease
Hypertension
Diabetes mellitus

CLINICAL MANIFESTATIONS

Pain, not relieved by rest or nitrates, possibly radiating to left arm, neck, and entire chest; pain may be less severe than in younger persons with myocardial infarctions or *may not occur at all*

Delirium
Dyspnea
Decreased blood pressure
Fluctuation in pulse rate (increase or decrease)
Moist, pale skin
Low-grade fever
Nausea and vomiting
Anuria as condition progresses

ADDITIONAL NURSING INTERVENTIONS
TO INCORPORATE INTO GENERIC CARE PLAN

• Support treatment plan:
   Oxygen to relieve hypoxic heart muscle
   Medications: analgesics (see Table 8-1), nitroglycerin (Table 7-5), antidysrhythmics (see Table 7-2), digitalis (see Table 7-4)

TABLE 7-5   Antianginals

Drug	Side effects	Nursing implications
Amyl nitrite (Vaporade)	Weakness, dizziness	Crush ampule in gauze or cloth; hold near nose for inhalation
		Do not use near fire or cigarettes (flammable)
		Encourage client to sit during administration
		Expect effect to last approximately 8 minutes
Nitroglycerin (Nitro-Bid)	Throbbing headache Dizziness Weakness Nausea, vomiting Skin rash	*Sublingual* Store properly to maintain potency Do not expose to light, heat, air Do not keep cotton in container Use nonmetallic container
		Expect rapid effect, less than 20 min duration
		If possible, use *before* exertion that could bring on angina (e.g., sexual intercourse, exposure to temperature extremes)
		Elderly clients might have difficulty producing enough saliva to moisten tablet

TABLE 7-5 Antianginals—cont'd

Drug	Side effects	Nursing implications
		Advise client to sit or lie while administered, because elderly are more sensitive to hypotensive effects of nitrates and can become dizzy and fall
		Burning sensation indicates drug is potent
		Repeat dose if necessary at 5- to 15-min intervals; administer no more than three doses
		Keep record of time taken and result
		Instruct client to seek medical assistance if three doses do not relieve attack
		Renew prescription every 6 mo
		Timed Release
		Take at least 1 hr before, 2 hr after meals
		Expect effect for 8-12 hr
		Topical
		Apply to hairless area for uniform absorption
		Rotate application sites
		Thoroughly remove residue from previous applications
		Expect action in 30 min, complete absorption in approximately 4 hr

Interactions
Effects increased by atropine-like drugs, tricyclic antidepressants.
Effects decreased by choline-like drugs (e.g., Mestinon, Prostigmin).
Propranolol can increase hypotensive effects of antianginals.

Lidocaine usually prescribed in lower doses because of age-related decrease in hepatic metabolism and increased risk of CNS side effects

Anticoagulants should be used with care because of increased risk of bleeding; dosage must be individualized and closely monitored (Table 7-6)

External or internal pacing

- Monitor vital signs, ECG, cardiac enzymes, hemodynamic parameters, arterial blood gases, intake and output, mental status:

TABLE 7-6   Anticoagulants

Drug	Side effects	Nursing implications
Dicumarol Heparin (reduced effectiveness in elderly) Phenindrone (more harmful side effects than most anticoagulants) Warfarin (usually started at one-half adult dose)	Bleeding; hemorrhage Unusual hair loss Itching Sores in mouth or throat	Observe for signs of blood loss: dizziness, headaches, bleeding gums or wounds, hemoptysis, vomiting coffee ground material, bloody or tarry stools, fever, chills, fatigue Keep skin moist Regularly examine oral cavity Have vitamin K available (antidote) Monitor prothrombin times closely; dosage adjustment may be necessary Ensure client is not taking salicylates (for arthritis, etc.) because 3 g or more can promote hemorrhage, suggest acetaminophen as alternative Review dietary intake for vitamin K–rich foods that can inhibit anticoagulant action (e.g., turnip greens, broccoli, cabbage, liver, spinach)

Interactions: all anticoagulants
Increase effects of phenytoin, hypoglycemic agents.
Decrease effects of cholestyramine.
Effects increased by alcohol, allopurinol, antibiotics (broad spectrum), chloral hydrate, chlorpromazine, colchicine, ethacrynic acid, mineral oil, phenylbutazone, phenytoin, probenecid, reserpine, salicylates, steroids, thyroxine, tolbutamide, tricyclic antidepressants.
Effects decreased by antacids, barbiturates, chlorpromazine, rifampin, vitamin K.

Change in pulse can indicate dysrhythmias.

Drop in blood pressure can be associated with shock.

Increased respirations may signify congestive heart failure or pulmonary edema.

Decreased arterial pH and P_{CO_2} levels can indicate metabolic acidosis.

Dyspnea, crackles (rales), and coughing can be signs of congestive heart failure.

Anuria can indicate worsening of condition.

Altered mental status and restlessness can indicate inadequate cerebral circulation.

- Promote rest to minimize strain on heart; use a bedside commode; support limbs with armrests and footstools.
- Encourage daily graded exercise and emphasize importance of avoiding physical and emotional stress.
- Maintain a comfortable environmental temperature.
- Prevent constipation to avoid additional strain on heart (see "Constipation," p. 117).
- Evaluate effects of medications.
- Spend time with client and encourage expression of concerns and feelings.
- Teach relaxation exercises.
- Educate client and family in realities of illness, its care and restrictions, including dietary alterations, smoking cessation, sexual activity; explain necessary life-style changes after recovery; provide encouragement to make those changes.

❖ Generic Care Plan:
ALTERED TISSUE PERFUSION

GENERAL INFORMATION

Altered tissue perfusion involves a decrease in nutrition and respiration at the cellular level caused by a decrease in capillary blood supply. Critical areas of concern among the elderly include cardiac, cerebral, and peripheral perfusion.

CAUSATIVE/CONTRIBUTING FACTORS

Interruption of arterial or venous flow

Cardiovascular disorders: atherosclerosis, arteriosclerotic heart/valvular disease, hypertension, congestive heart failure, pulmonary edema, hypervolemia or hypovolemia, aneurysms, varicosities

Blood dyscrasias: anemia, thrombus, embolus, transfusion reaction

Hypotension: septic shock, hypoglycemia, hyperglycemia, anaphylactic shock

Diabetes

CLINICAL MANIFESTATIONS

Tachycardia
Tachypnea, dyspnea
Angina
Altered mental status, restlessness
Peripheral
> Diminished peripheral pulses
> Claudication, flushing
> Change in skin color and temperature: cool, mottled, cyanotic, moist, shiny
> Edema
> Slow healing of cuts and sores, tissue necrosis

NURSING PROCESS

Assessment Considerations

- History of common precipitating factors, immediately preceding (i.e., the 5 E's: exercise, eating, exposure to cold, exertion, emotions)
- History of predisposing conditions: hypertension, phlebitis, arteriosclerotic disease, diabetes, obesity, cigarette smoking
- History of episodes of confusion or blackouts: duration, symptoms, deficits exhibited
- Mental status and ability to use and interpret language
- Vital signs, including three-position (lying, sitting, standing) blood pressure (see Box 7-3)
- Circulation; presence of visible, enlarged veins
- Peripheral edema
- Sensorimotor function
> Visual field, blind spots, blind area of visual field (homonymous hemianopsia or blindness in the same half of the visual field in both eyes)
> Swallowing problems
> Muscle weakness, drooping eyelid, drooling
> Asymmetry in strength, function, appearance

ECG changes (Figure 7-2) (Table 7-7)
Pain: degree, location, type, duration
Skin status

Goals

- Client is able to identify precipitating causes.
- Client demonstrates improved cardiac muscle perfusion.

Text continued on p. 176.

NORMAL SINUS RHYTHM (NSR)

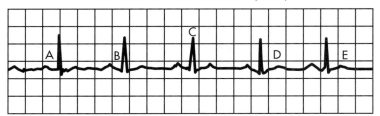

Each wave, as shown above, corresponds to a part of the heart cycle.

A. P wave	Represents contraction of the atria. Normally does not exceed 3 mm (3 small squares) in height or .12 second (3 small squares) in width. A larger P wave indicates atrial enlargement.
B. P-R interval	Represents time between start of atrial contraction to start of ventricular contraction. Normally does not exceed .20 second (5 small squares) in width. Prolonged P-R interval indicates cardiac damage.
C. QRS complex	Represents contraction of the ventricles. Normally Q wave should not exceed .04 second (1 small square) in width or exceed ⅓ the height of the QRS complex. An enlarged Q wave indicates an old coronary occlusion. An enlarged R wave indicates ventricular enlargement; a smaller R wave occurs when the heart is compressed by fluid.
D. S-T segment	A segment longer than 8 squares indicates hypocalcemia; a segment shorter than 4 squares represents hypercalcemia. An elevation of the segment above the baseline indicates myocardial infarction or pericarditis; a depression of the segment indicates reduced oxygen supply to the heart muscle.
E. T wave	Represents ventricular recovery. Normally should not exceed 10 mm (10 small squares) in height. A flat wave indicates a reduced supply of oxygen to the heart muscle; an inverted wave indicates myocardial infarction. An elevated T wave indicates elevated serum potassium.

FIGURE 7-2 Understanding the electrocardiogram. (From Hoeman S: *Rehabilitation/ restorative care in the community,* St Louis, 1990, Mosby–Year Book.)

TABLE 7-7 Common Cardiac Dysrhythmias

Dysrhythmia	Causes	ECG changes	Medical treatment
Premature ventricular contractions (PVC)	Myocardial infarction Heart disease Stress on normal hearts from effects of caffeine, smoking, or alcohol	Wide and irregular QRS complex	Some resolve without treatment Xylocaine if heart rate is over 60 beats/min Atropine if heart rate is slow
Premature atrial contractions (PAC)	Impulses originating outside sinus node Can occur in normal hearts	Abnormal P wave	Most resolve without treatment Quinidine when treatment is indicated
Paroxysmal atrial tachycardia (PAT)	Impulses originating outside sinus node Can occur in normal hearts	Abnormal P wave; perhaps indistinguishable from T wave of preceding beat Rate usually exceeds 100 beats/min	Stimulate right carotid sinus by using tongue depressor to initiate gagging for a few seconds Metaraminol or propranolol may be given Cardioversion (timed electric shock) should be used in serious cases
Sinus tachycardia	Impulses travel at faster rate because of overexertion, anxiety, fever, or other stress Can occur in normal hearts under stress	Rate exceeds 100 beats/min	Eliminate underlying cause

Sinus bradycardia	Digitalis or other drugs (secondary effect) Myocardial infarction Hearts conditioned by regular aerobic exercise	Rate less than 60 beats/min	Most resolve without treatment Atropine when treatment is indicated
Atrial flutter	Arteriosclerotic heart disease Rheumatic heart disease	Rate less than 60 beats/min	Most resolve without treatment Atropine when treatment is indicated
Atrial fibrillation	Arteriosclerotic heart disease Rheumatic heart disease	Irregular P waves Rapid rate	Digitalis (unless already taken) Cardioversion
AV block	Arteriosclerotic heart disease Myocardial infarction	First-degree AV block: longer P-R interval Second-degree AV block: some P waves occur without QRS complex Third-degree AV block: no relationship between P waves and QRS complex; slow rate	First degree: most resolve without treatment Second degree: atropine, isoproterenol, pacemaker Third degree: pacemaker; atropine or isoproterenol may be used until insertion
Ventricular tachycardia	Myocardial infarction (secondary complication)	P waves independent of QRS complexes Wider QRS complex Rapid rate	Xylocaine Cardioversion
Ventricular fibrillation	Myocardial infarction	Every wave and complex irregular	Life support Defibrillation (differs from cardioversion in that shock is not timed)

- Client is free from complications secondary to altered tissue perfusion.
- Client functions with maximum independence
- Client describes life-style changes necessary to improve condition.

Nursing Interventions
- Support prescribed treatment plan:
    - Antihypertensives (Table 7-8), antianginals (see Table 7-5), anticoagulants (see Table 7-6)
    - Dietary modification
    - Physical therapy or whirlpool
    - Surgery
- Monitor cardiovascular status and vital signs.
- Help client identify factors that interfere with good circulation and measures to avoid them, for example, avoidance of temperature extremes, prevention of angina attacks (prevention of attacks is important; recurrence over the years can cause myocardial fibrosis leading to myocardial weakness and congestive heart failure).
- Promote health practices that aid in promoting good tissue perfusion:
    - Weight reduction
    - Improved stress management
    - Proper diet
    - Smoking cessation
    - Moderate, regular exercise
    - Avoidance of constricting garments
- Encourage client to change positions slowly.
- Monitor for changes in mental status, sensorimotor functioning, headaches, or dizziness.
- Observe for signs of electrolyte imbalances.
- Observe for sudden onset of cyanosis, respiratory distress, diaphoresis, anxiety, or chest pain.
- Observe for ischemic signs from drug effects.
- Monitor vital signs and heart sounds on an ongoing basis and note changes in blood pressure; monitor postural blood pressure.
- Encourage client to rest and avoid activities that can increase the cardiac workload (e.g., straining when having a bowel movement); assist with development of an exercise program that slowly increases activity; ensure client performs or receives

TABLE 7-8 Antihypertensives

Drug	Side effects	Nursing implications
Clonidine hydrochloride (similar to methyldopa, most effective when given with diuretic)	Orthostatic hypotension	Monitor blood pressure
Guanethidine sulfate (one of most potent antihypertensives available, reduces systolic blood pressure more than diastolic)	Nausea, vomiting, anorexia, gastrointestinal disturbances	Advise client to change positions slowly
Methyldopa (for sustained hypertension)	Reduced WBC (particularly with propranolol) and platelet count	Monitor nutritional status and intake and output
Propranolol hydrochloride (slow reduction of blood pressure, therapeutic effect within 1 wk, wide variation in individual plasma levels, higher incidence of adverse reactions in uremic persons, more drowsiness than with other antihypertensives)	Impaired ejaculation	Ensure intake of adequate nutrients and fluid
Reserpine (action can continue for as long as 2 wk after discontinuation)	Depression, confusion, nightmares, hallucinations, psychotic behavior (particularly with reserpine and propranolol)	Observe for signs of infection, unusual bruises, bleeding
	Bradycardia (particularly with reserpine)	Ensure periodic blood work is evaluated
	Hepatitis (particularly with methyldopa)	Advise client that impaired ejaculation is related to therapy .
		Assess impact of sexual dysfunction on emotional well-being
		Monitor mental status
		Assess ability to participate in activities of daily living (ADLs), maintain safety, and intervene as necessary
		Reinforce reality
		Monitor vital signs
		Administer propranolol on full stomach, reserpine with meals
		Withdraw clonidine gradually to prevent rebound hypertension
		Protect client from cardiovascular effects of propranolol: patient with angina can develop myocardial infarction and die from sudden withdrawal,

Continued.

TABLE 7-8   Antihypertensives—cont'd

Drug	Side effects	Nursing implications
		extremities may feel cold because of reflex vasoconstriction; signs of shock and hypoglycemia can be masked

Interactions: all antihypertensives

Increase effects of barbiturates, insulin, oral antidiabetics, sedatives, thiazide diuretics, tolbutamide (by propranolol).

Decrease effects of antihistamines (by propranolol), antiinflammatory drugs (by propranolol).

Effects increased by phenytoin (by propranolol), thiazide diuretics (by guanethidine).

Effects decreased by amphetamines, antihistamines, tricyclic antidepressants.

Concurrent use of guanethidine with digitalis preparations can gradually reduce heart rate.

range-of-motion exercises three times daily; consult with physical therapist as necessary.

- Provide extra patience and time in caring for client who has experienced a sensory/motor deficit:

    Schedule longer periods of time for care activities.

    Talk with client during activities, even if client does not appear to understand.

    Keep client informed of current events.

    Use simple, straightforward directions and one-step instructions.

    Provide clocks, calendars, and familiar possessions.

    Anticipate emotional lability and depression; recognize that client may use profanity and be critical and that this should not be taken personally.

    Help family understand dynamics of condition and provide support.

- Initiate rehabilitation plans as early as possible; consult with physical, occupational, and speech therapists as necessary.

- Implement measures to prevent common complications (e.g., contractures, pressure ulcers, dependent edema, falls, accidents, choking, sensory deprivation, isolation, fatigue, unnecessary dependency).

For the client with altered peripheral tissue perfusion:

- Instruct client to monitor responses to walking and to stop if he/she experiences pain, fatigue, dizziness, or nausea.
- Teach client how to reduce pressure to pressure points by range-of-motion exercises, frequent change of positions, and not crossing legs.
- Ensure proper positioning to prevent contractures.
- Protect and instruct client in how to protect legs and feet from cuts, bumps, and pressure; reinforce that skin is highly susceptible to trauma, infection, and ulcerative lesions because of poor quality of circulation.
- Educate client in principles of good foot health (see Box 5-3):

  Wear footwear that offers good fit, support, safety, and comfort.

  Avoid walking barefoot or in slippers.

  Measure water temperature before washing or soaking feet (decreased sensations may prevent early detection that water is hot enough to burn).

  Wash feet with soap and water and dry thoroughly, particularly between toes; apply lotions to prevent skin dryness.

  Wear clean, well-fitting stockings, not tight enough to constrict or loose enough to wrinkle; avoid socks with dyes that bleed.

  Keep toenails trimmed straight across, even with edge of toes; do not dig under nail or cut off skin (many elderly have visual and mobility restrictions that limit ability to care for toenails; assess need for assistance; refer to podiatrist as indicated).

  Obtain podiatric care for corns, calluses, or other foot problems.

  Perform daily range-of-motion exercises to every joint.

  Give foot massages daily (unless thrombosis is present) to stimulate circulation, provide exercise, and promote relaxation:

  Clean and soak feet; dry thoroughly.

Warm hands, and apply lubricant to palms.
Cradle client's foot in both hands for a few seconds.
Make circular motions with the thumb over the sole of the foot.
Roll knuckles over the sole.
Rotate and gently pull each toe.
Knead the heel and ankle.
Massage the heel firmly.
Allow the client a period of relaxation afterward.

Evaluation
- Client identifies causative/contributing factors and changes life-style and activities accordingly.
- Client performs exercises regularly.
- Client has peripheral pulses that are equal and of good quality.
- Client is free from injury and complications related to condition and drug therapy.

Possible Related Nursing Diagnoses
Activity intolerance
Altered nutrition: more than body requirements
Anxiety
High risk for injury
Knowledge deficit
Self-care deficit
Sensory-perceptual alteration
Sexual dysfunction

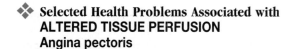

❖ Selected Health Problems Associated with ALTERED TISSUE PERFUSION
Angina pectoris

GENERAL INFORMATION

Angina pectoris is a condition associated with coronary artery disease that causes severe pain in the chest, often radiating from the left shoulder down the arm, as a result of ischemia of the heart muscle.

CAUSATIVE/CONTRIBUTING FACTORS

Atherosclerotic heart disease (obstructs coronary blood flow)
Severe aortic stenosis or insufficiency
Anemia
Hyperthyroidism
Tachycardia
Precipitating factors
      Physical exertion
      Cold weather
      Sexual activity
      Cigarette smoking
      Strong emotions
      Large, heavy meal

CLINICAL MANIFESTATIONS

Pain
      Mild to severe
      Usually lasting 3 to 5 minutes
      Located at middle or upper portion of sternum
      Tight, strangling, vicelike feeling around chest
      Radiates to neck, jaws, and shoulders
      More diffuse in many older persons
Apprehension
Weakness
Numbness in arms and hands

ADDITIONAL NURSING INTERVENTIONS
TO INCORPORATE INTO GENERIC CARE PLAN

- Assess the type of pain to determine if it is angina; anginal pain does not vary with breathing or body positions and is diffuse.
- Administer oxygen and medications as ordered and observe effects.
- Assist client to comfortable position and give support in calm manner.
- Instruct client to administer nitroglycerin properly (see Table 7-5).
- Reinforce importance of *preventing* anginal attacks, rather than just correcting them once they occur. Fibrotic scars can result

from attacks and increase risk of more serious myocardial disease.

Transient ischemic attack (TIA)

GENERAL INFORMATION

TIA refers to an impairment of cerebral blood flow that causes CNS dysfunction that lasts several minutes to several hours. Complete recovery usually occurs within 1 day, and there are no apparent residual effects nor any neurologic deficit between attacks. TIA is considered a warning signal and part of the stroke syndrome.

CAUSATIVE/CONTRIBUTING FACTORS

Coronary artery disease
Diabetes
Blood vessel spasms
Hypertension
Sudden reductions in cerebral blood flow (e.g., suddenly standing)
Anemia
Cigarette smoking

CLINICAL MANIFESTATIONS

Falling or collapse to floor
Aphasia
Diplopia or unilateral blindness
Amnesia (inability to recognize familiar persons or objects)
Numbness or complete loss of function in extremities; hemiparesis

ADDITIONAL NURSING INTERVENTIONS
TO INCORPORATE INTO GENERIC CARE PLAN

- Emphasize importance of adhering to treatment plan and seeking prompt medical care (TIA is a serious sign; risk of CVA increases with each TIA).

- Instruct client and family in emergency actions to take when an attack occurs.
- Aid family in developing mechanisms to monitor client (e.g., daily telephone call at mutually agreed-on time).
- Administer anticoagulants and other medications as prescribed. Teach safe use of prescribed medications and recognition of adverse reactions (see Table 7-6).
- Instruct client to change positions slowly (e.g., sit on side of bed 2 minutes before standing).
- Assist in identification and correction of causative/contributing factors.

Cerebrovascular accident (CVA)

GENERAL INFORMATION

A CVA is a severe, sudden decrease in cerebral circulation caused by either a thrombus (usual cause in the elderly) or a hemorrhage that results in a cerebral infarct. CVA, commonly known as a stroke, is a common neurologic cause of problems related to coordination and mobility and is the third leading cause of death in the elderly. The chances of CVA are increased with age, and men are more prone to experience and die from strokes than women. Symptoms can appear suddenly and profoundly or slowly and subtly and will vary depending on the area of the brain involved.

CAUSATIVE/CONTRIBUTING FACTORS

Hypertension
Atherosclerosis
Cardiac disease
Blood lipid abnormalities
Impaired glucose tolerance
Diabetes mellitus
Cigarette smoking

CLINICAL MANIFESTATIONS

Paralysis: hemiplegia, quadriplegia
Homonymous hemianopsia

Lightheadedness

Drop attack: complete muscular flacidity in lower extremities without alteration in consciousness

Spatial-perceptual deficits

Incontinence

Sensory loss

Impaired memory and judgment

Change in level of consciousness

Difficulty swallowing

Loss of control of emotions

Speech and language deficits

Anterior frontal lobe CVA

    Intact comprehension

    Altered speech, altered sentence structure

    Profanity used uncharacteristically and/or uncontrollably

    Impaired recognition of familiar objects

Posterior frontal lobe CVA

    Comprehension lost

    Confabulation or inappropriate grouping of words

ADDITIONAL NURSING INTERVENTIONS TO INCORPORATE INTO GENERIC CARE PLAN

- Be aware of cognitive deficits associated with right and left lesions:

  Right hemisphere lesion (left hemiplegia): no awareness of deficits, poor judgment, short attention span, inability to transfer learning, quick and impulsive movements, performance affected (not comprehension), not likely to regain prestroke capabilities

  Left hemisphere lesion (right hemiplegia): aware of deficits; impaired ability to read, write, speak; repetitive actions and speech; slow, cautious movements; comprehension affected; prestroke function more easily restored

- Review impact of illness and expected outcome with client and family:

  Current limitations and realistic expectation of improvement

  Type and anticipated duration of care-giving responsibilities

  Resources available to assist with care giving

- Recognize new physical and emotional demands placed on family and care givers; offer support.

- Promote highest level of self-care independence; obtain assistive devices; consult with occupational and physical therapy.
- Allow opportunities for ventilation of feelings; accept anger, depression, and other feelings as normal reactions to illness.
- Reinforce progress made and maintain an attitude of optimism and hope.
- Refer to the following nursing diagnoses for additional interventions:
    Self-care deficit
    Impaired mobility
    Impaired verbal communication
    Grieving
    Sensory-perceptual alteration: visual
    Impaired skin integrity
    Altered urinary elimination

Hypertension

GENERAL INFORMATION

Hypertension is a rise in systolic and/or diastolic blood pressure above the level judged normal for the individual. The Joint National Committee on the Detection, Evaluation, and Treatment of High Blood Pressure (in *Archives of Internal Medicine,* vol. 148, pp. 1023-1038, 1988) classifies hypertension as follows:

SYSTOLIC	DIASTOLIC	CLASSIFICATION
<140	<90	Normal
140-159	<90	Borderline systolic hypertension
≥160	<90	Systolic hypertension
	85-89	High normal diastolic
	90-104	Mild hypertension
	105-114	Moderate hypertension
	≥115	Severe hypertension

The types of hypertension are as follows:
    Primary (essential): No known cause, usually occurs between 30 and 50 years of age, accounts for majority of hypertension cases

Secondary: Caused by underlying primary disease, usually develops before 30 years of age or after 50 years of age

Benign: Slow, progressive rise in blood pressure

Malignant (accelerated): Abrupt, severe rise in blood pressure, diastolic greater than 130 mm Hg, papilledema present

CAUSATIVE/CONTRIBUTING FACTORS

Age-related changes causing increased rigidity of aorta, greater peripheral resistance

Obesity

Atherosclerosis

Anemia

Thyroid disease

Renovascular hypertension

Stress

Drugs (e.g., cold preparations, steroids)

CLINICAL MANIFESTATIONS

Asymptomatic: first clues to problem can be manifestations of underlying disease processes (e.g., TIA, mental status alterations)

Secondary hypertension can produce headache, flushing

Blood pressure above normal limits

ADDITIONAL NURSING CARE
TO INCORPORATE INTO GENERIC CARE PLAN

- Monitor vital signs, take blood pressure carefully on schedule as ordered (Box 7-3).
- Note symptoms and function in relation to documented blood pressure (e.g., if altered mental status is noted when blood pressure falls below a specific level, if headaches develop when blood pressure rises above a certain level).
- Ensure that antihypertensives are administered on time and consistently; monitor client for expected and adverse effects (see Table 7-8).
- Be aware of and monitor the following risks of hypertensive therapy:

BOX 7-3 Obtaining an Accurate Blood Pressure

- Help the client feel calm and comfortable:
  Avoid assessing blood pressure in extremely cold or hot environments (remember, the elderly are more sensitive to cold and may be uncomfortable in temperatures that do not bother nursing staff).
- Use a proper-fitting cuff:
  A proper cuff size is one in which the width is 40% the circumference of the arm.
  The length of the cuff should be sufficient to encircle the limb and, preferably, be twice the width of the cuff.
- Place the cuff on the limb snugly with the lower edge approximately 1 inch above the area where the stethoscope will be placed.
- Palpate systolic blood pressure before auscultating:
  Take the radial pulse (or popliteal if a leg reading is used) while the cuff is being inflated.
  Note the point at which the pulse is no longer palpable; this is the systolic blood pressure.
- Auscultate the blood pressure, listening for the five phases of sounds (called Korotkoff's sounds); phase 1 is the systolic blood pressure and phase 5 the diastolic pressure in adults:
  Phase 1: Point at which sounds are heard
  Phase 2: Period in which swishing sound is heard
  Phase 3: Period in which sounds are crisper and more intense
  Phase 4: Period in which sounds become muffled and have a soft quality
  Phase 5: Point at which sounds cease
- If possible, take blood pressure in sitting, lying, and standing positions (three-position blood pressure).
- Pulse strength may vary in elderly persons, making the blood pressure difficult to obtain. In such cases, readings may need to be estimated and this should be noted as such on the client's medical record.
- Take several readings to confirm blood pressure elevation; it may be useful to obtain a reading in the client's home, on a different day, reducing stress from the strange environment and medical examination.
- Record blood pressure, extremity used, and position of client during reading.

Persons with diabetes, with reduced renal function, with malnutrition, or on cardiac glycoside therapy have a higher risk of complications.

Depression can be caused or intensified by antihypertensives.

Antihypertensives can aggravate prostate problems.

Orthostatic hypotension is more likely in persons with poor cerebral blood flow.

Guanethidine sulfate must be discontinued several weeks before any anticipated surgery (vascular collapse, cardiac arrest can occur during anesthesia).

- Observe for episodes of hypotension; take blood pressure when client is supine and immediately again when client sits or stands upright.
- Maintain fluid and electrolyte balance.
- Educate client and family about hypertensive disease and management:

Asymptomatic nature

Need for effective stress management

Importance of regular medication (even if symptoms are absent)

Need for regular medical follow-up

Compliance with low-sodium, high-potassium diet, low in calories for weight control

Reduction of alcohol intake

Avoidance of smoking

Early recognition of complications such as congestive heart failure, myocardial infarction, changes in mental status, stroke, hypertensive retinopathy, renal disease

Varicose veins

GENERAL INFORMATION

Varicose veins are dilated elongated superficial veins. Most varicosities occur in the legs although they can occur anywhere in the body.

CAUSATIVE/CONTRIBUTING FACTORS

Age-related loss of vessel elasticity
Prolonged standing
Obesity
Multiparity
Hereditary weakness of vein wall
Chronic constipation (rectal varicosities)

CLINICAL MANIFESTATIONS

Visibly enlarged discolored veins
Leg cramps, aches
Fatigue
Edema
Dizziness when rising from lying position

ADDITIONAL NURSING CARE
TO INCORPORATE INTO GENERIC CARE PLAN

- Teach preventive measures regarding the importance of avoiding prolonged sitting or standing, constrictive clothing, and obesity.
- Stress the importance of improving circulation and avoiding complications such as thrombophlebitis and ulceration.
- Instruct client on proper use of support hose.
- Teach proper foot care, foot inspection, prevention of trauma to feet.
- Prepare for ligation and stripping of veins if surgery is planned.

Stasis ulcers of legs

GENERAL INFORMATION

Poor circulation in the legs can promote inflammation, leading to the development of lesions. Most stasis ulcers develop on the ankles.

CAUSATIVE/CONTRIBUTING FACTORS

Chronic venous insufficiency
Thrombophlebitis
Incompetent valves of the veins

CLINICAL MANIFESTATIONS

Pain may or may not be present; arterial ulcers are usually more painful than venous ulcers
Pigmentation, cracking appearance of the legs

Reddening of foot; foot may become pale when elevated
Leg edematous and cool to touch
Poor pulse in affected extremity
Dermatitis

ADDITIONAL NURSING CARE
TO INCORPORATE INTO GENERIC CARE PLAN

- Promote healing of ulcerated areas and keep free from infection and gangrene by the following measures:
    - Keep extremity elevated and warm
    - Keep bedclothes off injured area
    - Assist with ulcer debridement as directed, maintaining strict aseptic technique
    - Advise client to avoid scratching area
    - Implement and evaluate effectiveness of ordered treatments (e.g., Elastoplast or Unna's paste boot, antibiotics)
    - Assess for and reporting any signs of cellulitis (e.g., redness, edema, pain)
- Prepare client for surgery (e.g., ligation and stripping of veins) if planned.

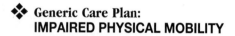

❖ Generic Care Plan:
IMPAIRED PHYSICAL MOBILITY

GENERAL INFORMATION

Impaired physical mobility is a state in which the person has some degree of difficulty or complete inability in moving purposefully in the environment. Movement restrictions may be imposed by medical order or may be the result of a physical or mental impairment.

CAUSATIVE/CONTRIBUTING FACTORS

CVA, nervous system disorders or injuries
Amputation
Fractures
Arthritis
Pain

Obesity
Depression, dementia
Fatigue
Dizziness
Medical conditions requiring enforced bed rest

CLINICAL MANIFESTATIONS

Muscle weakness, paralysis, or atrophy
Pain, inflammation of joints
Altered cognition, mood
Decreased level of consciousness
Incoordination, muscle twitching
Contractures, deformities
Limited range of motion

NURSING PROCESS

Assessment Considerations
- Range of motion in all joints
- Muscle strength
- Level of consciousness
- Cognition, motivation to participate in self-care activities
- Three-position blood pressure, vital signs
- Energy level
- Presence of pain
- Normality of structure and function of body parts
- Medications used
- Functional level: North American Nursing Diagnosis Association suggests coding level of independence as follows:

  0 = Complete independence
  1 = Requires use of equipment or device
  2 = Requires help from another person for assistance, supervision, or teaching
  3 = Requires help from another person and the use of equipment or device
  4 = Dependent, does not participate in activity

Goals
- Client increases level of mobility.
- Client is free from complications associated with immobility.
- Client uses mobility aids safely and properly.

Nursing Interventions

- Prevent immobility if possible; it takes approximately 7 days for the client to regain the function lost during 1 day of bed rest (Box 7-4).
- Position client properly, maintain good body alignment:
    Maintain body position as dictated by condition.
    Change position frequently (at least every 2 hours).
- Assess range of motion in every joint and initiate range-of-motion exercises (Table 7-9) unless contraindicated:
    Ensure body is in good alignment.
    Provide support above and below joint being exercised.
    Perform exercise slowly, smoothly, and gently for approximately five repetitions.
    Do not force joint past point of resistance or pain.
    Attempt to increase range of motion in restricted joints.

Text continued on p. 199.

BOX 7-4   Hazards of Immobility

CARDIOVASCULAR
Increased burden on heart
Orthostatic hypotension
Thrombus formation

RESPIRATORY
Increased effort necessary for
    breathing
Poor gas exchange
Hypostatic pneumonia

GASTROINTESTINAL
Decreased appetite
Constipation
Fecal impaction
Stress ulcers

SKIN
Decubitus ulcers

NEUROLOGIC
Sensory deprivation

MUSCULOSKELETAL
Bone weakening
Greater likelihood of bone fracture
Muscle atrophy
Contractures

URINARY
Stones
Urinary stasis
Urinary tract infection

SKIN
Decubitus ulcers

EMOTIONAL
Depression
Anxiety
Preoccupation with illness
Feelings of helplessness and
    hopelessness
Increased dependency
Exacerbation of latent neurosis,
    psychosis

Table 7-9 Range-of-Motion Exercises

Range of motion: maximum joint mobility (varies in each body joint)
- Flexion (bending)
- Extension (straightening)
- Adduction (moving toward side of body)
- Abduction (moving away from side of body)
- Internal rotation (turning inward at ball and socket joint)
- External rotation (turning outward at ball and socket joint)
- Circumduction (circular movement)
- Pronation (rotation down/toward the back)
- Supination (rotation up/toward the front)
- Inversion (turning in at other than a ball and socket joint)
- Eversion (turning out at other than a ball and socket joint)

Purpose of exercises
- Maintain joint motion and muscle strength
- Maintain functional capacity
- Prevent contractures

Types of exercise
- Active: client performs independently
- Passive: nurse performs for client
- Active with assistance: nurse and client work together

Be sure to provide adequate support for all involved joints when performing or assisting with range-of-motion exercises.

Joint	Normal range of motion
Shoulder (A, B, C)	Free straight arm motion from relaxed position at side, forward and overhead to 160-degree angle
	Free straight arm motion backward to 30-degree angle with body

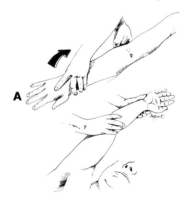

Shoulder in extended position. Flexion occurs as arm is lifted up and back.

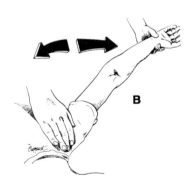

Sliding arm toward body produces shoulder adduction. Sliding arm away from body produces abduction.

Continued.

Table 7-9 Range-of-Motion Exercises—cont'd

Joint	Normal range of motion
	Free straight arm motion laterally to 160-degree angle

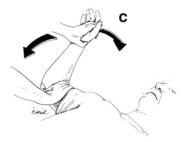

As forearm is brought down, internal rotation occurs at shoulder joint. As forearm is brought up and back, external rotation occurs.

Elbow (D, E)   From full-arm extension, hand should swing back to touch shoulder (160 degrees)

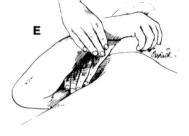

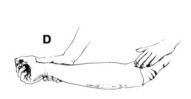

Elbow extended.   **Elbow flexed.**

Wrist (F, G, H)   From perpendicular with ground, wrist should rotate 90 degrees to each side
From parallel to ground, wrist should flex downward 80 degrees, upward 70 degrees

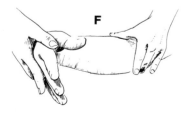

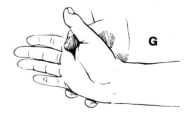

Wrist extended.   **Wrist flexed.**

Table 7-9 Range-of-Motion Exercises—cont'd

Joint	Normal range of motion
	From parallel with ground, wrist should move 10 degrees (thumbward), 60 degrees toward ulnar side

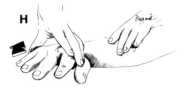

Lateral movement of wrist produces radial and ulnar deviation.

Finger (I, J, K)	Distal phalanx should flex 90 degrees (right angle with palm) and extend 30 degrees

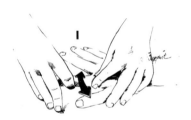

Fingers abducted away from midline and adducted toward midline (of hand).

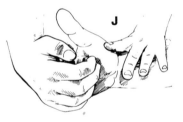

Fingers flexed as group into closed fist.

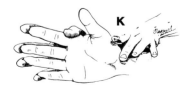

Finger extension is described as open fist.

Continued.

Table 7-9 Range-of-Motion Exercises—cont'd

Joint	Normal range of motion
Thumb (L, M, N)	Distal portion should bend 90 degrees (right angle) Proximal portion should bend 70 degrees

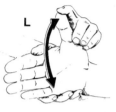

Thumb flexed toward and extended away from fourth digit.

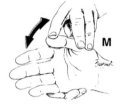

Thumb abducted and adducted in relation to other fingers.

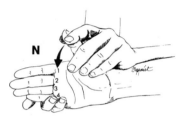

Thumb moved in opposition to base of each of other four digits.

Knee (O, P)	From prone position: 100-degree

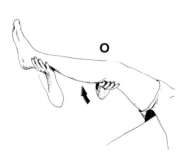

Movement of lower leg upward produces knee extension. Hip also in extension.

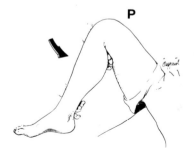

Knee and hip in position of flexion.

Table 7-9   Range-of-Motion Exercises—cont'd

Joint	Normal range of motion
Hip (Q, R, S, T, U)	From supine position, rising toward chin: 90 degrees with leg straight, 125 degrees with knee bent From prone position: 5-degrees backward extension From straight alignment with body: abduction of 45 degrees, adduction of 45 degrees

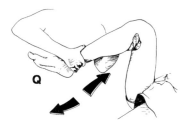

Caregiver can move hip in flexion by sliding leg back. Extension can be produced by sliding leg forward.

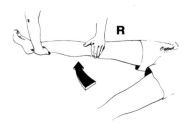

Moving leg away from midline of body abducts hip.

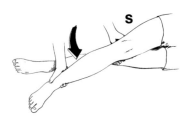

Moving leg toward midline of body and crossing over it adducts hip.

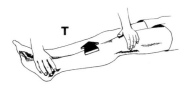

Rolling leg inward causes hip joint to rotate internally.

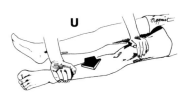

Rolling leg outward causes hip joint to rotate externally.

Continued.

Table 7-9   Range-of-Motion Exercises—cont'd

Joint	Normal range of motion
Ankle (V, W, X, Y, Z)	Dorsiflexion (toward head) of 10 degrees, plantar flexion (toward floor) of 40 degrees Inversion of 35 degrees, eversion of 15 degrees

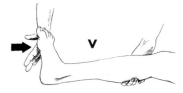

Pressure with palm of hand against ball of foot causes ankle dorsiflexion.

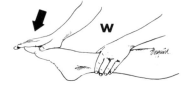

Pressure against top of foot causes ankle plantar flexion.

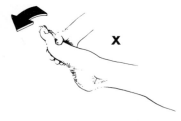

Turning foot inward produces ankle inversion.

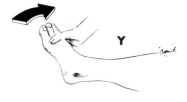

Turning foot outward produces ankle eversion.

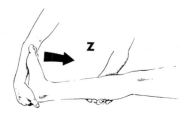

Heel cord stretching involves downward pull on heel cord and dorsiflexion of ankle.

Illustrations from Dittmar S: *Rehabilitation nursing: process and application,* St Louis, 1989, CV Mosby.

Incorporate range-of-motion exercises into routine activities (e.g., bathing, turning, walking) rather than making the program an isolated entity.

Regularly evaluate and record joint motion.

- Encourage appropriate exercises based on client's needs; consult with physical therapist as indicated.
- Use isometric, resistance, muscle-setting exercises if possible.
- Avoid positions that interfere with good circulation (Box 7-5).
- Ensure that client turns, coughs, and deep breathes at least every 2 hours.
- Ensure adequate fluid intake, high-fiber diet (unless contraindicated).
- Use massage, lotion, or protective devices as needed to protect skin integrity.
- Ensure that client obtains equipment and devices, as needed, and uses them appropriately (Box 7-6).
- Ensure client has easily accessible means to summon for help.

Text continued on p. 203

BOX 7-5   Proper Positioning

BED

No more than one pillow under head; do not flex neck.

Knees and hips straight: use sandbags or pillows to prevent external hip rotation; do not put pillow behind knees or otherwise cause flexion.

Ankles flexed at 90 degrees: use footboard or pillows if necessary.

Arms abducted from body and straight with slight flexion.

Hands flat; fingers open.

CHAIR

Head straight; avoid bending or dangling.

Trunk upright; do not bend or curve.

Arms and hands supported on armrest or tabletop; avoid dangling.

Hands flat; fingers open.

Hips and knees flexed; feet flat on floor or footrest, ankles flexed at 90-degree angle. If legs are kept straight with leg rest, keep ankles flexed at 90-degree angle.

BOX 7-6   Mobility Aids

CANE

Characteristics

- Assists balance by widening base of support; not intended for weight bearing
- Comes in a variety of styles
   Regular (straight): provides minimal assistance with balance
   Three- and four-point (quad): broader base of support, more cumbersome

Fit

- Length should approximate distance between greater trochanter and floor
- Elbow should be flexed slightly when cane rests 6 inches from side of foot

Use

- Use on unaffected side
- Advance when affected limb advances (i.e., if right leg is weak, the cane is held on the left and moved forward as the right leg steps) (Figure 7-3)
- Hold close to body; do not move forward beyond toes of affected foot
- All canes should have suction grips to prevent slippage on floor

WALKER

Characteristics

- Broader base of support; more stability than a cane
- Comes in a variety of styles
   Pickup: assists with weight bearing
   Rolling: pushed on wheels rather than lifted; reduces physical strain; often have seats to allow rest after several steps or propulsion from a sitting position

Fit

- Height equivalent to distance between greater trochanter and floor
- Elbows slightly flexed when hands on sides of walker

Use

- When weight bearing is allowed, advance walker and step normally
- When partial or no weight can be borne on one limb, thrust weight forward, then lift walker and replace all four legs on floor (Figure 7-4)
- Always use both hands when transferring from chair or commode; back walker to seat and use arms of chair or commode to assist in standing

WHEELCHAIR

Characteristics

- Used when client's disability prohibits other walking aids
- Should not be used for convenience or speed of client or staff

Continued on p. 202.

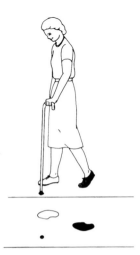

FIGURE 7-3 Ambulating with one cane or crutch. Shaded footprints and cane or crutch tips indicate where foot that bears weight is placed in each step. (This client has her right foot affected.) Client moves the cane forward, placing the tip on the floor just ahead of her unaffected, or stronger, leg and slightly out to the side of her foot. Then she takes one step forward with her affected leg. This brings the foot even with the cane or crutch. (From Hoeman S: *Rehabilitation/restorative care in the community,* St Louis, 1990, Mosby–Year Book.)

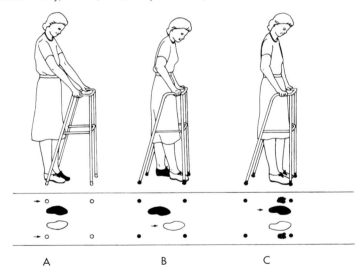

A   B   C

FIGURE 7-4 A walker assists many clients to ambulate. (This client has her right foot affected.) **A**, Client uses both hands to lift the walker and set it in front of her. **B**, She steps ahead with the affected foot and leg. **C**, She steps forward with the unaffected foot and stands. Her hand supports her weight on the walker. She repeats this process. (From Hoeman S: *Rehabilitation/restorative care in the community,* St Louis, 1990, Mosby–Year Book.)

BOX 7-6   Mobility Aids—cont'd

Fit
- Individually prescribed based on height, weight, limb use, arm strength, and self-propulsion capacity

Use
- Prepare environment for wheelchair use: widen doorways and toilet stalls; plan a functional furniture layout with no rugs; lower mirrors, telephones, drinking fountains, counters; install ramps
- Use special pads and cushions to reduce pressure damage; shift weight and reposition frequently
- Lock chair and remove footrests when transferring to/from

CRUTCHES
Characteristics
- Frequently difficult for older person to use because of inadequate upper body strength, arthritic hands, and balance problems
- Not as stable as other mobility aids

Fit
- Individually sized
- Length should be equivalent to 2 inches below axilla to point on floor 6 inches in front of client
- Hand bars placement crucial because hands should bear total weight
  Elbow should be flexed, wrist slightly hyperextended
  Axillary pressure can cause radial nerve paralysis

Use
- Tailor gait to client's needs; consult with physical therapist
- Use good posture and pay particular attention to foot position on affected side (walking exclusively on ball of foot or toes can cause footdrop)
- General rule when climbing stairs: stronger foot goes up first, down last (Figure 7-5)
  Upstairs: step up with stronger foot; bring crutches to that step; raise affected foot
  Downstairs: crutches to lower step; lower affected foot; follow with stronger foot
- Eliminate obstacles
  Waxed floors
  Throw rugs
  Extension cords
  Uneven surfaces
  Clutter

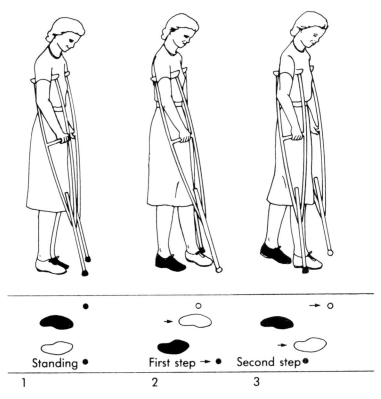

1	2	3
Standing ●	First step → ●	Second step ●

FIGURE 7-5 Shaded foot and cane or crutch tips are indicated for weight-bearing foot for each step. Two-point gait can enable many clients to become more active in ambulation. (From Hoeman S: *Rehabilitation/restorative care in the community,* St Louis, 1990, Mosby–Year Book.)

- Have frequent contact with client and promote socialization.
- If client is unconscious:
    Protect eyes from drying or accidental injury.
    Give oral hygiene every hour.
    Provide head rolls, and support feet.
    Ensure patent airway; have suction equipment available.

- Instruct client in proper way to fall to avoid serious injury:
  Fall toward affected side.
  Use unaffected side to raise self.
- Prevent and observe for complications from immobility (e.g., constipation, pressure ulcers, negative nitrogen balance).
- Recognize client's accomplishments in increasing mobility. Develop short-term goals to enable client to gain sense of accomplishment.

Evaluation
- Client demonstrates progressive increase in mobility.
- Client uses equipment and devices consistently and safely.
- Client is free from complications related to immobility.

Possible Related Nursing Diagnoses
Activity intolerance
Constipation
Fatigue
High risk for infection
High risk for injury
Impaired skin integrity
Incontinence, functional
Ineffective airway clearance
Powerlessness
Social isolation

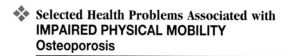

❖ Selected Health Problems Associated with
IMPAIRED PHYSICAL MOBILITY
Osteoporosis

GENERAL INFORMATION

Osteoporosis, the most prevalent metabolic disease of the bone, causes a reduction in the mineral and protein matrix of bones that results in diffuse reduction of bone density. The reduced bone density enables the bone to fracture under minimal stress. Osteo-porosis can be categorized as follows:

Primary osteoporosis: Most persons with osteoporosis have the primary form that is associated with menopause or an age-related bone loss that begins to be most pronounced after 70 years of age. The prevalence is higher in women.

Secondary osteoporosis: Although only a small portion of all osteoporosis results from secondary causes, it is the more likely form to occur in young women and men of all ages. A variety of factors can cause this type of osteoporosis, including hyperthyroidism, immobility, diabetes melli-tus, COPD, rheumatoid arthritis, and drugs (e.g., ste-roids, heparin, aluminum-based antacids, isoniazid, alco-hol, and tobacco).

CAUSATIVE/CONTRIBUTING FACTORS

Aging
Deficiency of calcium and protein in diet
Inactivity, immobility (causes high rate of bone resorption)
Estrogen/androgen deficiency
Race: more prevalent in whites and Asians
Low body weight
Chronic disease, e.g., diabetes mellitus, COPD, rheumatoid arthritis
Hyperthyroidism
Medications, for example, aluminum-based antacids, isoniazid, steroids
Cigarette smoking

CLINICAL MANIFESTATIONS

Asymptomatic usually until a problem occurs such as a fracture or collapsed vertebrae
Progressive loss of bone mass, spongelike appearance on x-ray, skeleton less dense
Weaker bones
Kyphosis
Reduced height
Back pain
Decreased spinal movement

ADDITIONAL NURSING CARE
TO INCORPORATE INTO GENERIC CARE PLAN

- Ensure client has received thorough examination to determine etiology; problems could be secondary to other disease, such as cancer.
- Review diet for calcium and protein intake; adjust diet to meet requirement. Ensure calcium intake of 1500 mg/day for post-menopausal women unless contraindicated.
- Advise menopausal and postmenopausal women to consult with their physicians regarding estrogen replacement.
- Consult with the physician and physical therapist regarding the use of supportive appliances and a bed board.
- Avoid immobility; assist with range-of-motion exercises. Encourage moderate weight-bearing exercises (e.g., walking).
- Teach client good body mechanics and ways to avoid strain.
- Protect limbs from fractures:
    Support limbs when moving client.
    Handle client's body with care.
    Pad side rails.
- Prevent contractures by proper positioning (see Box 7-5).
- Support client in weight reduction program if indicated.
- Carefully monitor urine output (hypercalcemia can result in kidney stones).

Fractured hip

GENERAL INFORMATION

After the sixth decade of life, hip fractures increase dramatically. Approximately one third of women and one sixth of men who live to 90 years old will experience a hip fracture. This fracture of the proximal end of the femur can be intracapsular (femur broken inside the joint) or extracapsular (femur broken outside the joint). The complications arising from a hip fracture can predispose the elderly to considerable disability as well as death (about 20% of hip fracture victims will die during the first year following the hip fracture). Falls are the most common cause of hip fractures in the elderly (Box 7-7).

BOX 7-7   Factors Contributing to Falls

AGE-RELATED CHANGES
Reduced visual acuity
Problems differentiating shades of
  same color (particularly greens,
  blues, violets)
Cataracts (cause glare to be more
  bothersome)
Poor vision in dimly lit areas
Less foot and toe lift during step
Altered center of gravity, balance
  lost more easily
Slower responses
Impaired muscle control
Poorer short-term memory
Orthostatic hypotension
Urinary frequency

**IMPROPER USE OF MOBILITY
AIDS**

MEDICATIONS
Can cause dizziness,
  lightheadedness,
  incontinence (e.g.,
  antihypertensives,
  sedatives, antipsychotics,
  diuretics)

UNSAFE CLOTHING
Poor-fitting shoes and socks
Long robes, pants legs

DISEASE-RELATED SYMPTOMS
Orthostatic hypotension
Incontinence
Reduced cerebral blood flow
Edema
Dizziness, weakness, fatigue
Brittle bones
Paralysis

Ataxia
Mood disturbances
Confusion

ENVIRONMENTAL HAZARDS
Wet surfaces
Waxed floors
Objects on floor
Poor lighting

STAFF-RELATED FACTORS
Use of restraints
Delays in responding to requests
Unsafe practices
Poor supervision of clients

From Eliopoulos C: Falls in the elderly, *Long-Term Care Educ* 1(1):3, 1990.

CAUSATIVE/CONTRIBUTING FACTORS

Falls
Stress on joint
Osteoporosis
Cancer metastasis to bone

CLINICAL MANIFESTATIONS

Affected extremity appears shorter, externally rotated, adducted
Pain
Inability to bear weight or move limb

ADDITIONAL NURSING INTERVENTIONS
TO INCORPORATE INTO GENERIC CARE PLAN

- Immobilize client after a fall has occurred and obtain an x-ray film immediately. Be aware that a fracture may not be apparent on a single x-ray film because of overlap or projection; anteroposterior and lateral views are necessary to make an accurate evaluation.
- Support the treatment plan, which can consist of traction, surgery (e.g., internal fixation, prosthesis), physical therapy, or occupational therapy.
- Control pain:
    Administer analgesics as prescribed; monitor effectiveness (see "Analgesics," p. 269).
    Use caution and gentleness in moving extremity.
- Begin rehabilitation as soon as possible:
    Assist client with range-of-motion and isometric exercises.
    Get client out of bed as soon as possible.
    Position client's body in proper alignment; prevent adduction and rotation of leg and hip flexion.
    Encourage self-care.
- Observe for and prevent complications:
    Thrombophlebitis or embolism
    Contractures
    Skin breakdown
    Shock or hemorrhage
    Infection
    Hip dislocation or refracture
- Provide emotional support:
    Client may fear permanent disability, dependency; help cli-

ent understand that new treatments and rehabilitation techniques hasten recovery.

Client may become discouraged during rehabilitative phase; set short-term goals, and acknowledge minor achievements in recovery.

Encourage client to be mobile; some clients become unnecessarily restricted in activities because of fear of falling and refracture.

- Be aware of and support physical therapy plan.

Arthritis

GENERAL INFORAMTION

Arthritis, or inflammation of the joints, is the leading chronic illness of the elderly. The well over 100 different types of arthritis can be categorized by cause as follows:

Cartilage degeneration: Develops when the cartilage breaks down and causes the ends of the bones to come in contact. Osteoarthritis, the leader in this category, increases in incidence with age and is the most common type of arthritis to affect the elderly.

Synovitis: Results from inflammation of synovial membrane, making joint red, tender, painful, and swollen. Rheumatoid arthritis is the most common example of this type and declines in incidence in late life.

Crystal arthritis (microcrystalline arthritis): Occurs because of small crystals (e.g., urate acid crystals) deposited in joint, leading to inflammation and pain as the body attempts to remove these crystals. Gout is the best known example of this type; it most often occurs in middle-aged men and postmenopausal women.

Joint infection: Develops when bacteria invade the joint and cause inflammation and discomfort. Most often, affected joints already have other forms of arthritis. *Staphylococcus* infections can be responsible for this type.

Enthesopathy: Results from inflammation of the tendons or ligaments, rather than the joint membrane. Ankylosing spondylitis is an example.

Other: Some forms of arthritis can result from joint injury or irritation, muscle inflammation, and other conditions.

CAUSATIVE/CONTRIBUTING FACTORS

Osteoarthritis
    Age-related degeneration of cartilage
    Trauma or stress on joint
    Obesity
Rheumatoid arthritis
    Cause unknown
    Thought to be autoimmune, genetic, or viral
Gout
    Overproduction or underexcretion of uric acid
    Thiazide diuretic therapy (inhibits excretion of uric acid)
    Heredity

CLINICAL MANIFESTATIONS

Osteoarthritis
    Slow, subtle progression of symptoms
    Joint discomfort, particularly on movement and weight bearing
    Joint stiffness
    Improvement of discomfort and stiffness with use of joint
    Altered posture and gait
    Crepitation (sound) with joint movement
    Heberden's nodes (bony growths) on distal joints of affected fingers
    Symptoms may increase during periods of overuse or weather changes
Rheumatoid arthritis
    Painful, red, swollen, tender, stiff joints
    Systemic symptoms: pain, anorexia, weight loss, fatigue, malaise
    Subcutaneous nodules over bony prominences
    Muscle atrophy of affected extremity
    Elevated sedimentation rate and erythrocyte count during attack
Gout
    Severe joint pain
    Swelling
    Redness, warmth of surrounding tissue
    Fever, malaise
    Elevated uric acid level
    Uric acid crystals in synovial fluid

ADDITIONAL NURSING INTERVENTIONS
TO INCORPORATE INTO GENERIC CARE PLAN

- Determine impact of disease on client's ability to fulfill ADLs:
  Consult with and support plans of occupational and physical therapists.
  Arrange for assistive devices as indicated.
  Encourage maximum independence.
- Determine range of motion of all joints (see Table 7-9).
- Help client to identify factors that trigger attacks such as stress, weather changes, specific foods; assist with development of lifestyle modifications to eliminate or minimize impact of factors.
- Control pain:
  Administer analgesics as ordered; instruct client in safe use of analgesics (see "Analgesics," p. 269).
  Apply heat or cold (according to client's response and physician's advice).
  Use braces and splints during acute episodes and at night if ordered.
  Prevent deformity.
- Control inflammation:
  Administer antiinflammatory agents as ordered (Table 7-10);
  Instruct client in safe use of antiinflammatory agents.
  Teach client how to limit stress to joints and to avoid physical and emotional stress.
- Discourage inactivity (Figure 7-6):

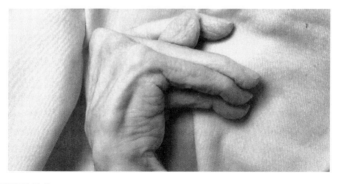

FIGURE 7-6 Severely contracted hands can result from lack of joint exercise. (From Castillo HM: *The nurse assistant in long-term care: a rehabilitative approach,* St Louis, 1992, Mosby–Year Book.)

TABLE 7-10 Antiinflammatories

General nursing measures
Observe for indications of bleeding.
Ensure periodic blood work is ordered and evaluated.
Protect from hazards related to impaired hearing and vision, dizziness; ensure communication is understood.
Monitor vital signs, mental status, intake and output, renal function.

Drug	Contraindications	Side effects	Nursing implications
Aspirin	Gastrointestinal disease, irritation Anticoagulant therapy	Gastrointestinal irritation increased blood values: SGOT, SGPT, bilirubin, alkaline phosphatase impaired/bone marrow depression Liver, kidney damage	Vitamin C can increase drug's effects
Adrenocorticosteroids	Cardiac, liver, or renal disease	Bone resorption, reduced formation of new bone Decreased glucose metabolism Fluid retention Increased risk of infection Aggravation of cataracts, glaucoma	Should be used with caution in elderly because of high risk of serious side effects Fracture potential is high so protect against injury Monitor blood glucose, intake and output, weight Observe for signs of infection Arrange for periodic ophthalmologic examinations

Drug	Contraindications	Side effects	Nursing considerations
Cholchicine	Cardiac, liver, renal or gastrointestinal disease	Gastrointestinal irritation Blood disorders	Preferred drug for treatment of gout Observe for signs of gastrointestinal bleeding
Fenoprofen	Asthma	Hemorrhage Visual disturbances Impaired hearing tinnitus Dizziness Renal failure (reversible)	Several weeks of therapy may be required for effects to be noted
Gold salts	Systemic lupus erythematosus Uncontrolled diabetes Severe hypertension Cardiac, liver, or renal disease	Pruritus, dermatitis Stomatitis Thrombocytopenia Agranulocytosis Bradycardia Nephritis Hepatitis Corneal ulcers Anaphylactic shock	Used to treat rheumatoid arthritis unresponsive to salicylate therapy May take several months to a year for full effects to be noted Note complaints of metallic taste that could indicate stomatitis Observe for skin irritation, itching; prevent skin breakdown
Oxyphenbutazone	Anticoagulant therapy Blood disorders Temporal arteritis	Bone marrow depression Hemolytic anemia Leukopenia	

Continued.

TABLE 7-10 Antiinflammatories—cont'd

Drug	Contraindications	Side effects	Nursing implications
	Dementia	Confusion	
	Gastrointestinal ulcers	Hypertension	
	Glaucoma	Visual disturbances	
	Cardiac, thyroid, hepatic, or renal disease	Hearing impairment	
		Hepatitis	
		Renal failure	
		Respiratory alkalosis	
		Metabolic acidosis	
Tolmetin	Asthma	Hyperthermia	
	Aspirin allergy	Prolonged bleeding	
		Dizziness	
		Sodium retention	
		Visual disturbances	
		Renal failure (reversible)	

Interactions: all antiinflammatories
Increase effects of oral anticoagulants, oral antidiabetics and insulin, penicillins, "sulfa" dugs.
Decrease effects of antihistamines (oxyphenbutazone), barbiturates (oxyphenbutazone), digitoxin (oxyphenbutazone), probenicid (aspirin), spironolactone (aspirin), tricyclic antidepressants (oxyphenbutazone).

Assist client in performing range-of-motion exercises to the point of pain but not beyond.
Involve client in care.
Consult with physical therapist about strengthening exercises.
- Consult with dietitian and assist client in making adjustments if low-purine or weight reduction diets are indicated.
- Provide support and counseling since awareness of progressive, disabling, deforming nature of some forms of arthritis can cause client to become depressed.
- Counsel client to avoid "fad cures" and to discuss all forms of treatment with physician before implementing.
- Prepare client for surgery if indicated:
    Arthroplasty: replacement of joint with prosthetic appliance
    Arthrodesis: fusion of bones
    Osteoplasty: removal of deteriorated bone from joint
    Osteotomy: excising bone to improve alignment

Parkinsonian syndrome

GENERAL INFORMATION

Parkinsonian syndrome is a progressive neurologic disorder that is the second most common neurologic disease of the elderly. It is characterized by muscle rigidity, akinesia, and involuntary tremor, with no impairment of intellectual ability. The incidence increases with age and occurs most frequently between the fifth and eighth decades of life. Most cases are *primary,* caused by Parkinson's disease. In some circumstances, parkinsonism can be *secondary,* in which it appears as a symptom of other problems.

CAUSATIVE/CONTRIBUTING FACTORS

Primary
    Parkinson's disease
    Paralysis agitans
Secondary
    Infection: encephalitis
    Drugs: neuroleptics, reserpine, methyldopa
    Tumors

Head trauma
Degenerative disorders of central nervous system
Arteriosclerosis
Toxins: occupational exposure to manganese, carbon dioxide

CLINICAL MANIFESTATIONS

Subtle onset of symptoms
Inability to control body movements (CNS impairment)
Tremor (decreases with purposeful movement), pill-rolling motion of fingers
Muscle rigidity
Slowness of movements
Masklike expression
Diminished eye blinking, presence of Myerson's sign (repetitive and synchronous blinking when forehead is tapped)
Shuffling, rapid gait with trunk leaning forward, lack of arm swing
Stooped posture
Muscle weakness
Drooling, difficulty swallowing
Slow monotonous speech
Increased appetite
Emotional instability (e.g., depression, anxiety)

ADDITIONAL NURSING INTERVENTIONS
TO INCORPORATE INTO GENERIC CARE PLAN

- Review impact of illness on daily living (e.g., feeding, swallowing, ambulation, hygiene, communication, toileting, safety).
- Administer antiparkinsonian medications to control symptoms:
    Administer on regular schedule.
    Eliminate pyridoxine (vitamin B_6) from diet when levodopa is administered (reduces effectiveness).
- Reinforce the need for regular medical follow-up; emphasize that although disease cannot be cured, its symptoms can be controlled or delayed with proper care.
- Expect emotional swings. Explain to family and care givers that this is a normal part of the illness that cannot be controlled.

- Respect client's intellectual status:
    Offer intellectually stimulating activities (e.g., reading, music) according to client's interests.
    Speak to client as adult.
    Be patient in allowing client to express self.
    Remind family and care givers of client's real intellectual abilities.
- Offer emotional support; reassure client and family that disease progresses slowly.
- Prevent stressful situations because tension and frustration will aggravate symptoms.
- Keep client involved with social and recreational activities.
- Compensate for self-care deficits:
    Teach alternate techniques for accomplishing tasks.
    Obtain occupational therapy advice.
    Introduce assistive devices and equipment.
    Perform tasks that client cannot.
    Maintain maximum independence.
- Protect client from hazards and complications such as choking and falls.
- Prevent contractures through range-of-motion exercises, massage, and proper positioning.
- Prevent falls (characteristic of disease is that when client is pushed, no attempt is made to stop the fall).
- Refer client and family to support groups.
- Also refer to the following care plans:
    Constipation
    Disturbance in self-concept
    Impaired physical mobility
    Impaired verbal communication

❖ Generic Care Plan:
ACTIVITY INTOLERANCE

GENERAL INFORMATION

Activity intolerance is a state in which the individual experiences an inability, physiologically or psychologically, to endure or tolerate an increase in activity.

CAUSATIVE/CONTRIBUTING FACTORS

Any factor that causes fatigue:
      Loss of endurance
      Advanced age
      Depression or lack of motivation
      Sedentary life-style
      Bed rest
      Sensory overload or deprivation
      Sleep disturbance
      Treatments or diagnostic studies
      Equipment that requires strength (walkers, etc.)
      Pain
      Impaired motor function
      Lack of incentive
Any factor that compromises oxygen transport:
      Cardiac: angina, dysrhythmias, congestive heart failure, myocardial infarction
      Respiratory: COPD, pneumonia, TB
      Circulatory: peripheral artery disease, anemia
Chronic diseases: renal, hepatitic, musculoskeletal, neurologic
Electrolyte imbalance
Hypovolemia
Malnourishment

CLINICAL MANIFESTATIONS

Weakness, fatigue
Pallor, cyanosis
Altered mental status
Vertigo
Inability to ambulate, turn in bed, perform self-care activities
Dyspnea, shortness of breath
Abnormal heart rate or blood pressure response to activity

NURSING PROCESS

Assessment Considerations
- History of activity level, recent changes
- Review of ADL and instrumental activities of daily living (IADL) (Tables 7-11 and 7-12)
- Presence of health problems that affect activity tolerance
- Vital signs

TABLE 7-11 Standards of Activities of Daily Living

	Level I independent	Level II requires mechanical assistance	Level III requires human assistance	Level IV totally dependent
Feeding	Able to eat without assistance	Needs special eating utensils	Needs food served and cut, packages opened, reminders to eat	Needs to be fed
Bathing	Able to get in and out of tub or shower and bathe all body parts	Needs grab bars, tub seats, adjusted faucet handles	Needs to be supported or lifted into tub or shower, back or other body part bathed	Needs complete bathing assistance
Dressing	Able to pick out appropriate garments and dress completely	Needs clothing and shoes modified with snaps or Velcro	Needs assistance with some garments and/or reminders of order to dress	Needs to be fully dressed
Continence	Able to completely control bowel and bladder elimination	Needs enemas, catheters	Periodically incontinent of urine or feces, needs to be reminded to toilet	Totally unable to control bowel or bladder elimination, catheterized
Toileting	Able to use toilet or bedpan and use proper related hygiene techniques	Needs bedside commode, bedpan, urinal	Needs assistance using commode or bedpan, wiping and cleansing after toileting	Unable to use toilet independently or clean self after elimination
Mobility	Able to walk and transfer from bed to chair	Needs cane, walker, crutch, wheelchair, brace, trapeze	Can walk, transfer, or use mobility aid with assistance	Totally unable to transfer, ambulate, or propel wheelchair

TABLE 7-12 Instrumental Activities of Daily Living Scale

Action	Score
A. ABILITY TO USE TELEPHONE	
1. Operates telephone on own initiative—looks up and dials numbers, etc.	1
2. Dials a few well-known numbers	1
3. Answers telephone but does not dial	1
4. Does not use telephone at all	0
B. SHOPPING	
1. Takes care of all shopping needs independently	1
2. Shops independently for small purchases	0
3. Needs to be accompanied on any shopping trip	0
4. Completely unable to shop	0
C. FOOD PREPARATION	
1. Plans, prepares, and serves adequate meals independently	1
2. Prepares adequate meals if supplied with ingredients	0
3. Heats and serves prepared meals or prepares meals but does not maintain adequate diet	0
4. Needs to have meals prepared and served	0
D. HOUSEKEEPING	
1. Maintains house alone or with occasional assistance (e.g., "heavy work–domestic help")	1
2. Performs light daily tasks such as dish washing, bed making	1
3. Performs light daily tasks but cannot maintain acceptable level of cleanliness	1
4. Needs help with all home maintenance tasks	1
5. Does not participate in any housekeeping tasks	0
E. LAUNDRY	
1. Does personal laundry completely	1
2. Launders small items–rinses socks, stockings, etc.	1
3. All laundry must be done by others	0
F. MODE OF TRANSPORTATION	
1. Travels independently on public transportation or drives own car	1
2. Arranges own travel via taxi but does not otherwise use public transportation	1
3. Travels on public transportation when assisted or accompanied by another	1
4. Travel limited to taxi or automobile with assistance of another	0
5. Does not travel at all	0

TABLE 7-12 Instrumental Activities of Daily Living Scale— cont'd

Action	Score
G. RESPONSIBILITY FOR OWN MEDICATIONS	
1. Is responsible for taking medication in correct dosages at correct times	1
2. Takes responsibility if medication is prepared in advance in separate dosages	0
3. Is not capable of dispensing own medication	0
H. ABILITY TO HANDLE FINANCES	
1. Manages financial matters independently (budgets, write checks, pays rent, bills, goes to bank), collects and keeps track of income	1
2. Manages day-to-day purchases but needs help with banking, major purchases, etc.	1
3. Incapable of handling money	0

From Lawton MP, Brody E: Assessment of older people: self-maintaining and instrumental activities of daily living, *Gerontologist,* 9:181, 1969.

- General physical status and strength
- Responses to activity (pre- and post-vital signs)
- Ability to move, stand, turn without assistance
- Causative factors (e.g., stress, psychologic, medications, lifestyle)
- Specific amount of activity tolerance and related symptoms (e.g., walks 100 feet without symptoms, becomes short of breath when walking 10 stairs)

Goals
- Client increases level of activity within individual limits of ability.
- Client expresses satisfaction with activity level.
- Client is free from complications related to activity intolerance.

Nursing Interventions
- Identify existing obtacles to activity and plan to reduce or eliminate these factors.
- Monitor vital signs before and after activity.
- Teach client and family the relationship between illness and inability to perform certain activities.
- Teach energy-saving techniques; consult with occupational and physical therapists as necessary.

- Plan care to include rest periods to reduce fatigue; have client participate in planning self-care activities.
- Administer analgesics as needed and promote comfort measures (see "Analgesics," p. 269)
- Protect client from injuries by giving assistance when needed and do not allow client to overexert self.
- Encourage a plan of exercise that involves a gradual increase in activity as tolerated.
- Ensure immobile client changes position regularly and puts all joints through range of motion at least three times each day.
- Provide protein supplements to regular diet if necessary.
- Teach client safety measures to prevent accidents and injuries (see "High Risk for Injury," p. 61).
- Increase client's incentive by setting realistic goals; provide positive reinforcement.

Evaluation
- Client is free from fatigue.
- Client tolerates increased activity levels.
- Client balances activity with rest periods.
- Client is free from injury and complications related to activity intolerance.

Possible Related Nursing Diagnoses
Altered nutrition: less/more than body requirements
Fatigue
High risk for impaired skin integrity
High risk for injury
Impaired physical mobility
Sleep pattern disturbance
Social isolation

❖ Generic Care Plan:
DIVERSIONAL ACTIVITY DEFICIT

GENERAL INFORMATION

Diversional activity deficit is the inability to occupy oneself in activities that pass time, entertain, or gratify. The individual experiences the environment as nonstimulating.

CAUSATIVE/CONTRIBUTING FACTORS

Physical limitations
Long-term hospitalization, institutionalization
Monotonous environment
Lack of motivation or interest
Retirement
Loss of significant others, pet
Inability to engage in usual hobbies, interests
Limited finances
Lack of transportation

CLINICAL MANIFESTATIONS

Verbal reports of "nothing to do," "I feel useless"
Yawning, inattentiveness
Restlessness, boredom
Withdrawn, hostile, lethargic behavior

NURSING PROCESS

Assessment Considerations
- Previous and current activity pattern, interests, hobbies
- Precipitating factors within environment
- Client's ability to participate in activity (physical, mental, socio-economic)
- Recent losses

Goals
- Client participates in at least one activity weekly.
- Client expresses interest in life.

Nursing Interventions
- Reduce or eliminate causative/contributing factors:
     Control pain.
     Obtain mobility aids, transportation.
     Refer for financial assistance.
- Offer activities that gave pleasure in the past.
- Encourage visitors; if client is in hospital or institutional setting evaluate benefit of placing in a semiprivate room for companionship.
- Introduce to new activities and offer them regularly.
- Refer client to activities and recreational and occupational therapists.

- Increase sense of self-worth by providing positive reinforcement.

Evaluation
- Client identifies and discusses feelings.
- Client participates in at least one new or previously enjoyed activity each week.

Possible Related Nursing Diagnoses
Activity intolerance
Anxiety
Disturbance in self-concept
Grieving
Impaired physical mobility
Pain
Social isolation

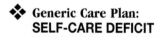

❖ **Generic Care Plan:**
  SELF-CARE DEFICIT

GENERAL INFORMATION

Self-care deficit exists when the individual is partially or totally unable to bathe, groom, dress, toilet, or feed self because of physical or mental factors.

Ill, disabled persons will have varying degrees of overall independence/dependence in ADL and IADL (see Tables 7-11 and 7-12). An individual may function at different levels for different tasks. For example, a client may be able to eat independently, bathe everything but the back, dress if helped with buttoning, walk, and use a toilet independently but will void on self unless reminded to go to the bathroom every 2 hours.

CAUSATIVE/CONTRIBUTING FACTORS

Immobility, impaired physical functioning
Trauma or surgical procedures
Impaired vision
Pain or discomfort
Perceptual/cognitive impairment
Musculoskeletal impairment

Neuromuscular impairment
Decreased strength and endurance

CLINICAL MANIFESTATIONS

Requires assistance with ADL or IADL (see Tables 7-11 and
  7-12)
Altered mental status
Impaired physical mobility

NURSING PROCESS

Assessment Considerations
• Functional capacity in feeding, bathing, dressing, grooming,
  toileting, moving, and maintaining continence (see Table 7-11)
• Causative/contributing factors (e.g., confusion, impaired sen-
  sory function, weakness, pain, missing limb, paralysis)
• Mental status or mood

Goals
• Client engages in ADL with maximum degree of independence.
• Client is free of complications associated with self-care deficits.

Nursing Interventions
• Preserve and use existing self-care capacity to maximize client's
  independence.
• Monitor intake and output, skin status, vital signs, bowel elim-
  ination.
• Identify specific causes of self-care deficit; adapt nursing inter-
  ventions accordingly (e.g., incontinence secondary to cognitive
  impairment would require different approaches from inconti-
  nence caused by a neurogenic bladder).
• Allow ample time for client to perform self-care activities.
• Gradually increase self-care responsibilities.
• Assist client in meeting ADL as necessary:
    Feeding: take food to client and set up tray, cut food, pour
      drinks, check in frequently to monitor amounts eaten and
      need for assistance.
    Bathing: lift in/out tub, draw water and regulate water tem-
      perature, bathe back and other hard-to-reach body parts,
      provide long-handled wash brush and soaped washcloth,
      use tub bench (Figure 7-7), remind client to bathe specific
      areas.

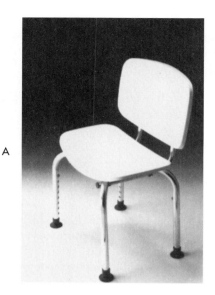

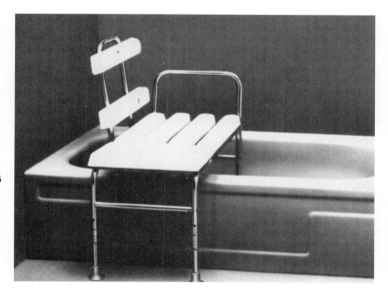

FIGURE 7-7 A, Adjustable-height tub bench. **B**, Padded adjustable transfer tub bench. (Courtesy Lumex, division of Lumex, Inc. From Hoeman S: *Rehabilitation/restorative care in the community,* St Louis, 1990, Mosby–Year Book.)

Dressing: retrieve clothing from closet and select outfits for client, lay out clothing in appropriate order and encourage client to dress self, provide special clothing (e.g., Velcro instead of buttons) and special equipment (e.g., zipper aid) to ease the process of dressing, remind to dress, help with specific garments, and/or dress client completely if necessary.

Toileting: provide bedside commode/bedpan/urinal/elevated seat (Figure 7-8), ensure easy access to bathroom, keep bathroom light on at night, assist in walking to bathroom or transfer to commode, determine elimination pattern and remind client to toilet accordingly and clean self after toileting, help with cleaning if necessary, check for incontinence, provide protective briefs or appliances as needed, provide change of clothing and assist client to clean skin after incontinence.

Mobility: see "Impaired Physical Mobility," p. 190.

- Protect client from injury.
- Refer to physical therapy, occupational therapy, and self-help groups as necessary.

Evaluation
- Client increases self-care capacity.
- Client eliminates or compensates for self-care deficits with adaptive devices or care giver assistance.
- Client fulfills all ADL.
- Client is free from complications.

Possible Related Nursing Diagnoses
Altered nutrition: less than body requirements
Disturbance in self-concept
High risk for fluid volume deficit
High risk for impaired skin integrity
High risk for injury
Impaired home maintenance management
Impaired physical mobility

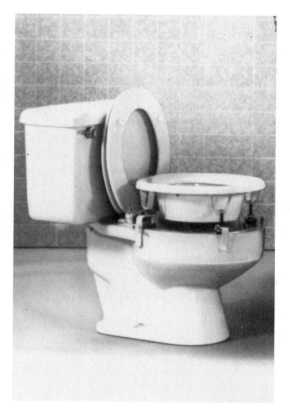

FIGURE 7-8 Elevated toilet seat. (Courtesy Lumex, division of Lumex, Inc. From Hoeman S: *Rehabilitation/restorative care in the community,* St Louis, 1990, Mosby–Year Book.)

❖ **Generic Care Plan:**
IMPAIRED HOME MAINTENANCE MANAGEMENT

GENERAL INFORMATION

Impaired home maintenance management occurs when an individual experiences difficulty in maintaining a safe, growth-promoting home environment. The environment includes one in which physiologic and psychosocial needs can be met.

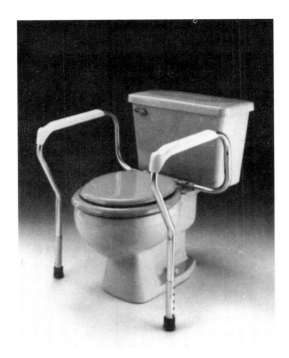

FIGURE 7-8—cont'd Adjustable toilet safety rails.

CAUSATIVE/CONTRIBUTING FACTORS

Chronic debilitating disease
Injury or illness to client or family or household member
Limited finances
Cognitive, motor, or sensory deficits
Inadequate support systems or community resources
Lack of knowledge or skill in home maintenance management
Reduced coping capacity

CLINICAL MANIFESTATIONS

Verbal statements by client or family of having difficulty maintaining self at home

Poor hygienic practices
    Infections, infestations
    Unwashed linens, dishes, clothes
    Disorderly, unclean surroundings
Unavailable support system
Overtaxed, stressed family members
Financial crisis
Evidence of inappropriate environmental temperature, lack of bathroom or kitchen facilities, lack of privacy, malfunctioning utilities

NURSING PROCESS

Assessment Considerations
- Functional capacity, physical limitations
- Mental status or mood
- Presence of health problems
- Family or support system
- Housing layout, size, condition, safety
- History of household management

Goals
- Client maintains clean, safe home environment.
- Client obtains and uses resources to enable competent home maintenance management.

Nursing Interventions
- Teach client home maintenance management skills (e.g., food handling, disinfection, insect control).
- Assist in locating resources that can improve environment as needed (e.g., improved lighting, extermination, correction of plumbing or electrical problems).
- Ensure environmental temperature that ranges between 70°F to 75°F.
- Educate family to the availability of aids for home care (Box 7-8).
- Arrange for assistance through homemaker aide, volunteer, family member, home-delivered meals; social service agencies can offer guidance on available resources, financial aid.
- Explore alternatives with client and family (e.g., relocation, obtaining live-in companion or occasional housekeeper).

BOX 7-8   Aids for Home Care*

Hospital bed
Trapeze bar
Overbed table
Hydraulic lift
Lift chair
Bedpan/urinal
Bedside commode
Bedding protectors/underpads
Protective undergarments/incontinence briefs
Bed-wetting alarm
Wheelchair/walker/cane
Grab bars, safety seats, nonslip strips for bathtub
Side arms, guard rails, and adjustable-height seats for toilets
Flotation cushions
Telephone amplifier and dial enlarger
Easy grip utensils
Vacuum-type feeding cup
Clothing with Velcro fasteners
Medical-emergency alarm systems

---

*Available through Sears Home Health Care Specialog or local medical supply stores.

- Discuss the option of nursing home placement for impaired, dependent elderly.
- Reassess self-care capacity of client and care givers on a regular basis:

    Their physical and mental status may change.
    New expenses, repairs, security problems may arise.

Evaluation

- Client functions adequately and safely at home.
- Client is free from injury and infection related to environmental conditions.

Possible Related Nursing Diagnoses

High risk for infection
High risk for injury
Ineffective individual/family coping
Self-care deficit

❖ **Generic Care Plan:**
SLEEP PATTERN DISTURBANCE

GENERAL INFORMATION

Sleep pattern disturbance is a disruption of sleep time that causes the client discomfort or interferes with the client's desired life-style.

Sleep pattern changes with age. Degenerative changes in the CNS cause older adults to sleep lighter and awaken more easily. Stage IV sleep (Box 7-9) is decreased or absent in the elderly.

BOX 7-9   Stages of Sleep

STAGE I NREM (NON–RAPID EYE MOVEMENT) SLEEP
Light sleep, individual can be easily awakened; eyes roll from side to side; heart and respiratory rates slightly decrease; will reach next stage within several minutes if left undisturbed; if sleep is interrupted during any of the other stages, the cycle will return to this stage

STAGE II NREM SLEEP
Higher state of relaxation; sleep remains light and easily broken; heart and respiratory rates continue to decline, as does body temperature; eyes tend to be still

STAGE III NREM SLEEP
Early phase of deep sleep; body processes continue to slow; muscles relax; sleeper requires moderate stimulation to arouse

STAGE IV NREM SLEEP
Deepest stage of sleep; extreme relaxation; typically, sleeper reaches this stage in 20 to 30 minutes and spends about 30 minutes in this stage; decreased vital signs and body movement; considerable stimulation required to awaken sleeper; deprivation can cause depression, apathy, lethargy; this stage greatly diminished with age and may be absent in some older adults

REM (RAPID EYE MOVEMENT) SLEEP
Deepest sleep level; decreased tonus of head and neck muscles; increased, possibly irregular vital signs; electroencephalogram (EEG) resembles stage I; sleepers drift into REM from stage IV about once every 90 minutes, four or five times each night; can be interrupted by amphetamines, alcohol, barbiturates, or phenothiazine derivatives; deprivation can result in irritability, anxiety, acute psychotic episodes

---

Older persons' sleep is more often interrupted by nocturia, muscle cramps, and noise. After interruption, older adults require more time to return to sleep. Less total night sleep is required (5 to 7 hours usually are sufficient), but the frequency of naps increases.

CAUSATIVE/CONTRIBUTING FACTORS

Pain
Stress
Anxiety or fear
Insufficient daytime activity
Nocturia
Unfamiliar environment
Change in usual sleep or activity pattern
Interruptions (e.g., noise, cold environment, treatments)
Illness-related symptoms (e.g., paroxysmal nocturnal dyspnea, coughing, orthopnea, pain)
Alzheimer's disease (reduces REM sleep and NREM sleep, stages III and IV); Parkinson's disease (decreases REM sleep and increases total wake time); medications (e.g., alcohol and antidepressants decrease REM sleep, nightmares can be caused by some antihypertensives, antiarrhythmics, and levodopa)

CLINICAL MANIFESTATIONS

Difficulty falling asleep
Daytime fatigue, yawning, nodding
Nocturia
Awakening in the middle of the night
Complaints of wakefulness

NURSING PROCESS

Assessment Considerations
- Sleep and rest history, usual bedtime and waking
- Activity pattern
- Sleep inducers
- Environmental preferences (e.g., temperature, lights, noise)
- Number of trips to bathroom during night
- Medications used
- Emotional stability
- Energy level

Goal
- Client is able to sleep 6 to 8 hours nightly uninterrupted.

Nursing Interventions
- Assist with diagnosis and treatment of underlying problem.
- Accommodate client's unique sleep habits by offering snacks, leaving radio on, and providing extra blankets.
- Assist client in nonmedical means of bedtime relaxation such as baths, backrubs, warm milk, and passive exercise.
- Encourage activities during the day that promote sleep such as exercise, ventilation of feelings, proper diet, sensible medication, and treatment schedules.
- Avoid interruptions when client is falling asleep (e.g., keep noise level down, do not flash lights, avoid bumping bed).
- Observe client's sleep for frequent periods of awakening, breathing problems, and restlessness.
- Discuss with client possible underlying fears, conflicts, and unresolved problems that may contribute to sleeplessness.
- Avoid performing procedures unnecessarily during the night.
- When hypnotics are absolutely necessary, use those least disruptive to the normal sleep cycle (e.g., flurazepam, diazapam, chlordiazepoxide).

Evaluation
- Client sleeps at least 5 hours nightly.
- Client reports feeling rested on awakening.

Possible Related Nursing Diagnoses
Activity intolerance
Anxiety
Fatigue
Pain

RECOMMENDED READINGS

Ancoli-Israel S: Epidemiology of sleep disorders. In Roth T, Roehrs T, editors: *Clinics in geriatric medicine*, Philadelphia, 1989, Saunders.

Cunha BA, Gingrich D, Rosenbaum GS: Pneumonia syndromes: a clinical approach in the elderly, *Geriatrics* 45(10):49, 1990.

Ettinger WH: Joint and soft tissue disorders. In Abrams WB, Berkow R, editors: *The Merck manual of geriatrics*, Rahway, NJ, 1990, Merck Sharp and Dohme Research Laboratories.

Gebhart TN: Fractures. In Abrams WB, Berkow R, editors: *The Merck manual of geriatrics,* Rahway, NJ, 1990, Merck Sharp and Dohme Research Laboratories.

Gleckman RA: Pneumonia: update on diagnosis and treatment, *Geriatrics* 46(2):49, 1991.

Herrera CO: Sleep disorders. In Abrams WB, Berkow R, editors: *The Merck manual of geriatrics,* Rahway, NJ, 1990, Merck Sharp and Dohme Research Laboratories.

Hoch CC: Sleep in old age. In Baines EM, editor: *Perspectives on gerontological nursing,* Newbury Park, CA, 1991, Sage.

Holm K, Walker J: Osteoporosis: treatment and prevention update, *Geriatr Nurs* 11(3):140, 1990.

Horowitz LN, Lynch RA: Managing geriatric arrhythmias, *Geriatrics* 46(3):31, 1991.

Kedas A, Lux W, Amodeo S: A critical review of aging and sleep research, *West J Nurs Res* 11:196, 1989.

Kinzel T: Managing lung disease in late life: a new approach, *Geriatrics* 46(1):54, 1991.

Kovach CR, Shore B: Managing a tuberculosis outbreak, *Geriatr Nurs* 12(1):29, 1991.

Leibovitch ER: Congestive heart failure: a current overview, *Geriatrics* 46(7):22, 1991.

Levine JM: Leg ulcers: differential diagnosis in the elderly, *Geriatrics* 45(6):32, 1990.

Miller M, Gottleib SO: Preventive maintenance of the aging heart, *Geriatrics* 46(7):22, 1991.

Moser M: Physical changes in the elderly: are they clinically important in the management of hypertension? *Geriatrics* 44(10):4, 1989.

Present D, Shaffer B: Disease associated with fracture: detection and management in the elderly, *Geriatrics* 45(3):48, 1990.

Schron EB, Friedman LM: Cardiovascular options for the 1990s, *Geriatr Nurs* 11(4):187, 1990.

Taylor JL: Overcoming barriers to blood pressure control in the elderly, *Geriatrics* 45(2):35, 1990.

Webster JR, Kadah H: Unique aspects of respiratory disease in the aged, *Geriatrics* 46(7):31, 1991.

8

 Cognitive and Perceptual
Processes

Appropriate and effective interaction with the elements of one's environment depends on adequate cognitive and perceptual processes. Through perceptual processes, the body uses its sensory organs to receive and carry messages from the external world. Cognitive processes then interpret those messages, using information retrieved from the memory.

For the most part, these processes operate without our conscious thought or effort. They are taken for granted until there is a problem with their function.

With age, a variety of sensory changes can cause misperception of one's world. Such changes include the following:

- Poorer vision: presbyopia; narrowing of visual field; decreased pupil responsiveness to light; decrease in pupil size; increased light perception threshold; yellowing of lens, leading to distorted perception of green, violet, and blue colors; slower dark-light adaptation; diminished corneal sensitivity
- Hearing loss: presbycusis; increased auditory reaction time
- Less taste sensitivity, especially for sweet and salty flavors
- Diminished olfaction
- Increased threshold for pain and touch
- Altered proprioception
- Decreased ability to differentiate temperatures

These changes can distort the messages received by the body.

Normally, cognitive function (memory, orientation, judgment, language, and calculation abilities) is not lost with age; however, there is an increase in diseases characterized by cognitive impairment. Such diseases include dementias, cerebrovascular accident (CVA), and cancer. As a result, many risks to physical, emotional, and social well-being arise.

Health education is extremely important to aging individuals. It enables them to clarify and accommodate common age-related changes to sensory function, identify symptoms of cognitive and sensory impairments, and learn and use skills and resources to compensate for deficits.

❖ Generic Care Plan:
ALTERED THOUGHT PROCESSES

GENERAL INFORMATION

Altered thought processes occur when there is a disruption in mental activities, including thought, language competency, reality orientation, problem solving, judgment, and comprehension. The client may appear bewildered, perplexed, or disoriented and behave and speak inappropriately.

Older adults can experience altered thought processes as an acute event in response to a disruption of the body's physical or emotional homeostasis; this is known as _delirium._ Deliriums differ in origin, treatment, and recovery potential from _dementias,_ which are irreversible, chronic alterations in thought processes.

CAUSATIVE/CONTRIBUTING FACTORS

Sleep deprivation
Psychologic conflicts, depression
Drugs, substance abuse
Emotional trauma
Environmental changes (relocation, hospitalization)
Head injuries, brain tumors
Metabolic disturbances
Nutritional deficiencies, fluid and electrolyte imbalances
Infections

Conditions causing inadequate cerebral oxygenation (chronic obstructive pulmonary disease [COPD], hypotension)
Also see discussions of dementia (p. 244) and delirium (p. 247)

CLINICAL MANIFESTATIONS

Misinterpretation of environment
Reduced attention span, easy distractability
Disorientation to time, place, person
Decreased ability to grasp ideas
Changes in remote, recent, or immediate memory
Impaired ability to make decisions, reason, calculate, conceptualize
Difficulty understanding or using language, expressing self
Hallucinations, delusions
Altered sleep patterns, sundowners' syndrome (Box 8-1)
With delirium: altered level of consciousness
Altered laboratory values

NURSING PROCESS

Assessment Considerations

- Mental status examination
- Extent of impairment in orientation, memory, thinking ability, attention span
- Speech, ability to understand and use language
- Changes in behavior
- History of problem: onset, precipitating factors, symptoms, pattern
- Potential causative/contributing factors: medications, dietary habits, presence of infections, sensory deprivation, stress
- Laboratory tests: blood, urine, cerebrospinal fluid
- Diagnostic tests: Electroencephalogram (EEG), echocardiogram (ECG), computed tomography (CT), magnetic resonance imaging (MRI), single photon emission computed tomography (SPECT)

Goals

- Client experiences correction of underlying cause if possible.
- Client demonstrates normal mental function.
- Client performs self-care activities with maximum independence.
- Client is free from injuries.

BOX 8-1   Sundowners' Syndrome

WHAT IT IS

Agitation, disorientation, wandering, and general worsening of behavior as evening approaches ("after the sun goes down")

CAUSE

Not fully understood, although occurs most frequently in persons with impaired cognitive function; contributing factors include recent admission to a health care facility, recent relocation within a health care facility, change in circadian rhythms (persons with sundowners' have higher oral temperatures and lower blood pressures in afternoon), dehydration, sensory overload or deprivation, use of restraints, and conditions that interrupt sleep

HOW TO HELP

Reduce pronounced transition from day to night by turning on lights before evening and using night-lights; frequently check on client; place familiar objects and personal possessions within client's view; provide afternoon activity; ensure adequate fluid intake; offer toileting assistance; use touch therapeutically

---

Nursing Interventions

- Assist in eliminating or minimizing underlying cause (e.g., correction of fluid and electrolyte imbalance, discontinuation of drug, improvement of nutritional status).
- Be aware that confusion and restlessness may be worse at night; monitor client to prevent injuries; provide frequent contact and reassurance. Prevent sundowners' syndrome (see Box 8-1).
- Promote orientation to reality (Box 8-2):
    Clarify misperceptions.
    Offer orientation to person, place, and time throughout the day.
    Use memory aids and simple one-step instructions.
    Use clocks and calendars.
    Do not support or ridicule delusions.
- Ensure client's right to make decisions is not violated; offer explanations and assistance as needed; refer to legal counsel if client's competency is in question and guardianship is needed; ensure care givers are aware of advance directive and durable power of attorney.
- Ensure medications are administered appropriately; elicit help from family member or friends if necessary.
- Administer antipsychotic medications as prescribed (Box 8-3);

BOX 8-2   Reality Orientation

Reality orientation is a process that helps keep clients with moderate-to-severe memory loss, confusion, and/or disorientation in touch with the immediate world around them.

- Encompasses all aspects of environment, all hours of the day
- Emphasizes stability in the environment, routine, staff
- Includes frequent, patient reminders of person, time, place
- Uses environmental aids
    Clocks
    Calendars
    Individual color schemes
    Reality boards
- Offers immediate feedback and rewards for success
- Is implemented with respect and patience
    Simple, honest responses to questions
    Calm voice
    Reality-oriented conversations
    Sensitive, caring attitude

GROUP CLASSES

- Select four to six clients with similar levels of cognitive function; prepare them individually for the class.
- Assemble group in a quiet, nondistracting environment.
- Put group at ease (offer refreshments, conversation, etc.).
- Identify each client by name; indicate verbal and nonverbal pleasure at his/her attendance.
- Speak to each client individually; compliment or otherwise express interest in each as a person.
- Review reality board
    Today is: Tuesday
    The date is: March 9
    The weather is: Cool and windy
    Our next meal is: Lunch
    The next holiday is: Easter
- After reviewing the board, ask the group questions related to the board: "What day is it, Mr. Smith?", "Mrs. Kent, what kind of weather do we have today?"
- Reward good responses immediately; correct but do not overreact to or dwell on errors.
- Offer a simple activity
    Singing a song
    Picking out pictures of specific items from a magazine
    Exercising
    Planting flowers
- With advanced groups, conduct current events or special topic discussions.
- Limit the group to 15 to 20 minutes to accommodate limited attention spans.
- It may be useful to assess the mental status of group members at the first session and periodically thereafter to note any changes that may occur.

document specific client behaviors (e.g., yelling, slapping, asking same question repeatedly) when giving antipsychotic medications; monitor effect of drug on controlling observable behaviors (Figure 8-1).
- Monitor nutritional status, intake and output.
- Evaluate self-care capabilities and compensate as needed.
- Determine factors that precipitate violent behavior and attempt to prevent them; protect client and others from violent and inappropriate behaviors of client.
- Avoid overstimulation.
- Control noise and lighting.
    Limit traffic flow in environment.
    Use relaxation techniques (e.g., soft music, warm baths, back rubs).

Evaluation
- Client is oriented to person, place, and time.
- Client speaks and behaves appropriately.
- Client is free from injury or secondary complications.

BOX 8-3   Antipsychotic Drugs

Antipsychotic drugs can have profound effects in older adults. They can produce sedation, hypotension, and anticholinergic and extrapyramidal symptoms.

ANTICHOLINERGIC SYMPTOMS

Dry mouth	Restlessness	Short-term memory loss
Constipation	Fever	Hallucinations
Urinary retention	Confusion	Agitation
Blurred vision	Disorientation	Picking behaviors
Insomnia		

EXTRAPYRAMIDAL SYMPTOMS

Parkinsonism: tremors; postural unsteadiness; rigidity of muscles in limbs, neck, and trunk; pill-rolling motion with fingers; shuffling gait
Akinesia: decrease in spontaneous movement
Dystonia: holding neck or trunk in rigid, unnatural position, such as turned to one side or hyperextended
Akathisia: inability to sit still
Tardive dyskinesia: thrusting movements of tongue; lip smacking, puckering, or chewing movements; abnormal limb movements

Continued.

BOX 8-3   Antipsychotic Drugs—cont'd

Commonly prescribed antipsychotic drugs and their risk of side effects are listed following:

Generic Name	Brand Name	Sedation	Hypo-tension	Anti-cholinergic symptoms	Extra-pyramidal symptoms
Acetophenazine	Tindal	Mild	Mild	Moderate	Mild
Chlorpromazine	Thora-zine	Marked	Marked	Marked	Mild
Fluphenazine	Prolixin	Mild	Mild	Mild	Marked
Haloperidol	Haldol	Minimal	Minimal	Mild	Marked
Loxapine	Loxitane	Mild	Mild	Moderate	Moderate
Mesoridazine	Serentil	Marked	Moderate	Mild	Minimal
Molindone	Moban	Mild	Mild	Moderate	Moderate
Perphenazine	Trilafon	Mild	Mild	Moderate	Moderate
Thioridazine	Mellaril	Marked	Marked	Marked	Mild
Thiothixene	Navane	Mild	Mild	Mild	Marked
Trifluoperazine	Stelazine	Mild	Mild	Mild	Marked

NURSING IMPLICATIONS

- Use antipsychotic medications only when absolutely necessary and for the management of **specific** target symptoms. The physician's order should describe the specific behaviors for which the drug should be used.
- Ensure that the smallest possible therapeutic dosage is administered initially. If desired results are not seen, the dosage can be gradually increased.
- Regularly assess client's behavior, intake and output, and side effects.
- Help client and care givers understand that several weeks of therapy may be needed before the effectiveness of the drug is noticed.
- Consult with the physician to reduce the dosage and discontinue the drug as soon as clinically feasible.

Possible Related Nursing Diagnoses

Anxiety
High risk for fluid volume deficit
High risk for infection
High risk for injury
High risk for violence
Impaired verbal communication
Impaired social interaction

CLIENT'S NAME   ROOM #

ANTIPSYCHOTIC DRUG USE FLOW CHART

Date:							
MEDICATION: List target behaviors for each drug prescribed and for each document frequency of occurrence:							
ORIENTED — D							
E							
N							
% MEAL CONSUMED — B							
L							
D							
PULSE							
TEMPERATURE							
RESPIRATIONS							
BLOOD PRESSURE							
TIMES SLEEPING/NAPPING							
ADVERSE EFFECTS (Use letter that corresponds to sign/symptom) D = dizziness, V = vision disturbance, R = restlessness, H = hallucinations, A = agitation, T = tremors, U = difficulty urinating, M = muscle rigidity, L = lip smacking, E = tongue protruding, G = shuffling gait, F = pill-rolling motions with fingers, B = frequent blinking (*state others*)							

FIGURE 8-1 Antipsychotic drug use flow chart.

Self-care deficit
Sensory-perceptual alteration
Sleep pattern disturbance
Social isolation

❖ Selected Health Problems Associated with ALTERED THOUGHT PROCESSES: Dementia

GENERAL INFORMATION

Dementia is a general, irreversible, progressive deterioration of mental function caused by organic factors. Dementias affect approximately 4 million Americans, most of whom are over 70 years of age.

Alzheimer's disease is the most common form of dementia. This condition begins as a mild impairment in cognitive function that can be mistakenly attributed to being busy, eccentric, or absentminded. As the cognitive impairment continues, the ability to meet basic needs and protect oneself from harm becomes jeopardized. Many times, only the shell of the individual remains, as aimless wandering, meaningless chatter, decreased emotions, and dependency on others for basic needs increasingly predominate. Alzheimer's disease is devastating for the entire family unit. Family members need guidance and support as they confront the disease-related changes of their loved one, assume care-giving responsibilities, and make difficult decisions concerning the welfare of themselves and the Alzheimer's victim. The affected individual needs continued attention to basic needs, protection from hazards, preservation of dignity, and the communication of caring that is important to all human beings.

CAUSATIVE/CONTRIBUTING FACTORS

Alzheimer's disease: senile plaques, neurofibrillary tangles, granulovacuolar degeneration; exact cause not known, some relationship to:

   Genetic predisposition: positive family history increases risk of developing; similarities between Alzheimer's disease and Down's syndrome in that choline acetyltransferase is reduced in both disorders

Abnormal protein structure: victims accumulate proteins not normally found in the brain, abnormally high beta amyloid level

Reduced level of enzyme choline acetyltransferase. Interferes in synthesis of acetylcholine

Multiinfarct dementia (ischemic cerebral lesions)

Alcoholism (Wernicke's encephalopathy)

Pick's disease: narrowing of frontal and temporal lobes, extreme shrinkage of localized cortical areas, reduction in neurons in affected areas

Jacob-Creutzfeldt disease: believed to be transmitted through slow virus

Parkinson's disease (one half of Parkinson's victims develop dementia)

Huntington's disease: inherited disease that begins in young adulthood, dementia usually appears in late stage

HIV-related dementia: more than 50% of acquired immune deficiency syndrome (AIDS) victims develop rapidly progressing dementia

Hydrocephalus, brain tumors

Trauma

Heavy metal toxicity

CLINICAL MANIFESTATIONS

Onset gradual, progressive

Decline in intellectual function
   Memory disturbance
   Disorientation
   Decreased conceptual thought
   Impaired abstract thinking

Changes in affect
   Easily frustrated
   Anxiety
   Depression
   Lability

Volatile coping reactions
   Anger, agitation, sullenness
   Evasiveness, withdrawal
   "Catastrophic reactions": agitation, irritability when faced with overwhelming situation

Sundowners' syndrome (see Box 8-1)

Decreased attention span
Preoccupation with self
Amnesia
Suspicion, paranoia
Difficulty in communication, aphasia
Confabulation
Delusions (often paranoid)
Excessive orderliness
Impaired judgment and decision making
Poor awareness of surroundings/environment
Apraxia, impairment of learned movements
Self-care deficits (later stages)
Brain changes detected on scans, EEG

ADDITIONAL NURSING INTERVENTIONS TO INCORPORATE INTO GENERIC CARE PLAN

- Provide a safe, structured environment:
    Control environmental stimuli.
    Place chemicals, medications, and potentially ingestible items out of client's sight.
    Create a defined, limited area for walking and wandering.
    Install bells or alarms on doors to signal client's exit.
    Color code or use consistent symbol (e.g., a flower) on client's room and possessions.
- Consider client's anxiety, attention deficit, and intellectual limitations when scheduling activities (Figure 8-2); several short sessions may be preferable and more effective than a single long one.
- Monitor intake and output:
    Encourage client to eat.
    Provide easy-to-eat foods and increase caloric intake when client is restless and wandering.
    Regularly remind client to toilet.
    Monitor client's weight:
        Weigh at least monthly.
        Weigh daily if client has lost more than 5% of total body weight in last 30 days.
- Provide consistency to schedule, procedures, care givers.
- Guide client in and monitor activities of daily living.
- Give simple, clear directions, one at a time; break tasks into simple steps.

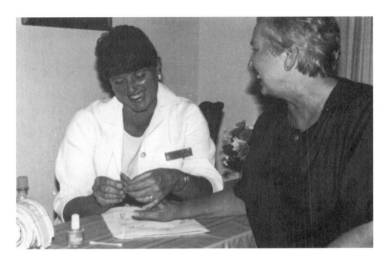

FIGURE 8-2 Clients with altered cognition may require assistance with basic grooming. (From Castillo HM: *The nurse assistant in long-term care: a rehabilitative approach,* St Louis, 1992, Mosby.)

- Orient to reality; do not foster misperception.
- Use consistency in approaches and care.
- Examine client's body regularly (e.g., during baths) for signs of problems such as skin breakdown, rashes, cuts, bruises, masses. Remember that client is less able to identify and communicate these problems independently.
- Be alert to nonverbal clues of problems (e.g., restlessness, appetite changes, behavior changes, rubbing body part, restricting limb usage, wincing).
- Promote maximum independence.
- Continuously reassess status and adjust care accordingly.
- Offer support to family members; refer to local Alzheimer's Disease and Related Disorders Association.

Delirium

GENERAL INFORMATION

Delirium is an acute confusional state marked by defective perception, impaired memory, and a rapid succession of disoriented and unconnected ideas, often accompanied by illusions and hallucinations. A characteristic feature is an altered level of consciousness, ranging from states of stupor to hypervigilance.

Delirium typically is precipitated by exogenous conditions. Once the underlying cause is treated, the person usually returns to a normal state of functioning.

CAUSATIVE/CONTRIBUTING FACTORS

Impairment of cerebral circulation, hypoxia
Malnutrition, dehydration
Metabolic imbalance
Prolonged sleep deprivation
Decreased cardiac, respiratory, renal function
Burns
Reaction to surgery
Infection
Alcohol or drug toxicity
Hyperthermia

CLINICAL MANIFESTATIONS

Change in level of consciousness: hypervigilance to coma
Combativeness, restlessness, agitation
Insomnia, nightmares, disturbed sleep-wake cycle
Tachycardia
Increased blood pressure
Apprehension, irritability
Confusion, disorientation
Auditory or visual hallucinations
Illusions, delusions

ADDITIONAL NURSING INTERVENTIONS
TO INCORPORATE INTO GENERIC CARE PLAN

- Assess and intervene promptly, because condition is reversible and treatment can prevent permanent damage.
- Use treatment appropriate to cause, and note results when treatment is instituted.
- Provide a quiet environment and adequate lighting to facilitate orientation.

- Establish and adhere to a consistent routine.
- Maintain a stable, moderate room temperature (approximately 75°F).
- Prevent injury by client to self and others.

Schizophrenic disorders

GENERAL INFORMATION

Schizophrenic disorders are psychotic states characterized by disturbed thinking, withdrawal from reality, regression, and poor interpersonal relationships. Some researchers think that the stresses experienced by many older adults or a lifetime's accumulation of stresses may intensify pathologic character traits of schizoid personalities. The specialized care needed by the schizophrenic person requires the involvement of a psychiatrist since ineffective management can reduce functional ability and increase the client's risk of institutionalization.

CAUSATIVE/CONTRIBUTING FACTORS

Cause unknown, may be the result of:
    Poor family relationships
    Traumatic experiences
    Maladaptive coping
    Chemical imbalance

CLINICAL MANIFESTATIONS

Auditory and visual hallucinations
Illogical thinking
Incoherence
Disorganized thoughts
Flat, inappropriate, or silly affect
Disorganized or peculiar behavior
Poor hygiene, inappropriate dress
Social withdrawal and isolation
Excited motor activity inconsistent with environmental stimuli

ADDITIONAL NURSING INTERVENTIONS
TO INCORPORATE INTO GENERIC CARE PLAN

- Maintain a stable environment and routine by limiting client's contact with unfamiliar people; introduce new staff members and explain their functions as necessary.
- Help reduce misperceptions by correcting sensory problems (vision or hearing deficits) and avoiding harsh lighting or shadows, unidentified sounds.
- Promote social contact, and include client in reality-oriented activities.
- Prevent complications (e.g., malnutrition, poor hygiene) resulting from abnormal behaviors.
- Develop a positive and trusting relationship, and provide a safe and secure environment.
- Divert focus from delusional material to reality, and avoid confirming or feeding into delusion.
- Encourage client to express negative and positive emotions.
- Be familiar with various antipsychotics used to control agitation, delusions, hallucinations, and psychotic symptoms (see Box 8-3).
- Be aware that antipsychotic medications are used to help make the client more receptive to other forms of therapy, not to substitute for other therapies.
- Ensure that proper dosages are prescribed for the older client:
    One third to one half of normal adult dosage is usually prescribed.
    Begin with lower dosage, and gradually increase to point of maximum benefit and least side effects.
- Observe response to medication carefully, because individual responses vary (see Box 8-3).
- Recognize extrapyramidal side effects of medications (e.g., dyskinesia, involuntary motor movement resembling Parkinson's).
- Ensure client does not consume alcohol or other central nervous system (CNS) depressants while taking an antipsychotic.

Paranoia

GENERAL INFORMATION

Paranoia is a mental disorder characterized by the presence of suspiciousness and delusions. The person often believes others are out to get him or her (e.g., the FBI, police). A delusion is a fixed belief (false) held with conviction despite evidence to the contrary. When the symptoms are relatively mild, the condition is known as paranoid personality. Paranoid reactions can occur in organic, alcoholic, and other mental illnesses. Paranoid states can be associated with age-related losses (e.g., sensory deficits) that increase feelings of anxiety, powerlessness, and suspiciousness, or they can be associated with dementia.

CAUSATIVE/CONTRIBUTING FACTORS

Organic illness, mental illness
Dementia
Alcohol, drug abuse
Sensory deficits contributing to misperceptions of environment
History or threat of being victimized

CLINICAL MANIFESTATIONS

Suspiciousness, mistrust of others
Delusions of persecution or grandeur
Low self-esteem
High anxiety level
Hostility toward others
Self-imposed isolation
Delusions of having thoughts controlled, messages broadcast to
  brain, extraordinary powers

ADDITIONAL NURSING INTERVENTIONS
TO INCORPORATE INTO GENERIC CARE PLAN

- Establish presence and onset of delusional thoughts; when did unusual behavior become noticeable to others? to client?
- Question about specific events surrounding delusional thoughts: they may be a reaction to or an exaggeration of a real threat (e.g., fears of personal harm are well founded in clients who live in high crime area).
- Obtain a thorough physical, mental, and social assessment to rule out other possible causes (e.g., organic disorders, trauma, hearing deficit).
- Make a special effort to establish rapport.
- Realize that paranoid people desperately need warmth and

understanding; do not be put off by client's distrust and accusations.

- Recognize client's unimpaired intellectual capacity and resentment of being "talked down to."
- Arrange for and support psychotherapy.
- Be honest with client by not supporting delusions, but avoid trying to convince client otherwise; this only reinforces the defense and belief systems.
- Avoid arguing with client about delusions, because the paranoid person cannot be rationally persuaded from fixed beliefs.
- Avoid power struggles and arguing with client, because it increases anxiety and hostility.
- Prevent isolation of client, and focus on reality situations in the environment.
- Monitor impact of paranoia on general health (e.g., nutritional status [fear of poisoning may interfere with food intake], hygienic practices [client may refuse to bathe and change clothes because of belief that someone is watching]).

❖ Generic Care Plan:
IMPAIRED VERBAL COMMUNICATION

GENERAL INFORMATION

Speech and language problems include disorders that interfere with the production, comprehension, or expression of words. Speech and language are not synonymous. *Speech* is the mechanics of producing words; *language* is the comprehension and expression of ideas. People can have speech problems, language problems, or a combination of both. Effective nursing care depends on knowing the specific cause of the speech or language problem. Early rehabilitative measures can decrease psychologic trauma and promote normal function and independence.

CAUSATIVE/CONTRIBUTING FACTORS

Anatomic defects
Motor disorders that interfere with word formation
Neurologic disturbances that limit comprehension, expression
Altered cerebral circulation

Cognitive deficits that alter word organization, interpretation

Hearing deficits that decrease or distort received words

Ethnic or cultural identity that causes linguistic differences between client and nurse

CLINICAL MANIFESTATIONS

Aphasia: loss of language function, usually caused by problems within the central nervous system; can be *expressive,* in which there is an inability to communicate thoughts verbally or in writing because of a motor problem; *receptive,* with an inability to comprehend language because of a sensory problem; or *mixed,* a combination of expressive and receptive

Dysphasia: impaired use of words; can be *receptive,* in which the client cannot understand words; or *expressive,* in which the client cannot organize words correctly or use the right name for a person or object

Dysarthria: problem with articulation because of poor motor control of the lips, tongue, and/or pharynx; client will use correct word but have difficulty pronouncing it

Paraphasia: a mild form of aphasia in which one word is substituted for another (e.g., clock for watch)

May appear confused, disoriented

NURSING PROCESS

Assessment Considerations

- Lip, tongue motion
- Soft palate symmetry, rise
- Vocal cord movement
- Gag reflex, swallowing
- Respiration
- Articulation (speed and quality)
- Appropriateness of language
- Hearing
- Simple tests of language difficulty

    Show five everyday objects and ask the name of each (e.g., pen, cup, book, comb, paper clip).

    Put the objects aside and then have client point to each as you name it.

    Ask client to repeat several simple sentences.

    State an expression or truism and ask the client to explain

its meaning (e.g., "People in glass houses shouldn't throw stones. . .").

Have client repeat "ma, ma, ma" (tests motor control of lips); "la, la, la" (test tongue); "ga, ga, ga" (tests pharynx); note distortions and slurring.

Goals
- Client is able to communicate needs and comprehend what is being said.
- Client communicates in a clear and appropriate manner.

Nursing Interventions
- Refer to speech therapist; support speech therapy plan.
- Determine the client's actual deficits and capabilities.
- Describe the speech or language impairment to the client (if possible), the family, and all care givers.
- Treat the client like an intelligent adult; realize that an inability to form words does not necessitate shouting or talking as if to a child.
- Keep client oriented by describing current events, introducing care givers, and explaining activities.
- Maximize existing strengths by using visual cues and assistive devices such as flash cards and communication boards containing common words for the client to point to; pen and paper; synthesizers and other assistive devices as recommended by the therapist.
- Be patient and accepting of the client's impairment; allow the client time to process words.
- Promote socialization and diversion; encourage family to visit; talk to client during care activities.
- Refer to support groups (e.g., Lost Chord Club) as appropriate.

Evaluation
- Client communicates effectively.
- Client participates in activities of daily living to maximum degree possible.

Possible Related Nursing Diagnoses
Anxiety
Disturbance in self-concept
Fear
High risk for injury

Impaired social interaction
Sensory-perceptual alteration
Social isolation

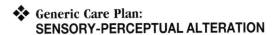

❖ **Generic Care Plan:**
SENSORY-PERCEPTUAL ALTERATION

GENERAL INFORMATION

Sensory-perceptual alterations exist when the usual and accustomed sensory stimuli are not experienced or recognized accurately. The individual experiences a change in the amount, pattern, or interpretation of incoming stimuli as a result of physiologic, sensory, motor, or environmental disruptions. The age-related declines in sensory organ function predispose the elderly to major impairments in recognizing and interpreting sensory stimuli.

Presbycusis is a sensorineural hearing loss experienced with age and is a common problem of the elderly. It is characterized by a loss of the ability to hear high-frequency sounds; as the condition progresses, middle- and low-frequency sounds are difficult to hear. The loss affects the ability to hear consonants more than vowels. Conductive hearing losses can accompany presbycusis, further distorting incoming sounds.

Visual problems are common in the elderly. Most older adults experience presbyopia (farsightedness), yellowing of the lens (which distorts the perception of low tone colors—blues, greens, violets), opacity of the lens (cataract formation), and slower light-dark adaptation.

Taste buds are lost with age, primarily affecting sensations for salty and sweet flavors.

Tactile sensations are decreased; many elderly are less able to feel pain and pressure.

Olfaction is reduced with age.

CAUSATIVE/CONTRIBUTING FACTORS

Age-related changes to sensory organs
Neurologic disease (e.g., CVA, glaucoma, neuropathies)
Musculoskeletal problems (e.g., paralysis)
Recurrent ear, eye, or upper respiratory infections

Ear wax accumulation
Medications
    Sedatives
    Tranquilizers
    Ototoxic drugs: salicylates, streptomycin, kanamycin
Environmental factors
    Change in environment
    High or multiple noise stimuli
    Poor lighting
Physical or social isolation
Trauma

CLINICAL MANIFESTATIONS

Impaired ability to see, hear, taste, smell, or feel
Inappropriate responses or behaviors
Disorientation, confusion
Anxiety, fear, apathy
Social isolation, withdrawal
Suspiciousness
Visual or auditory hallucinations
Restlessness, sleep disturbances
Inattention
Inappropriate responses or behaviors
Unusually loud speech
Requests to have words repeated
Cocking head in the direction of the "good" ear
Paranoia (believe others are talking or whispering about them
    behind their backs)
Frequent injuries

NURSING PROCESS

Assessment Considerations
- History of symptoms client is experiencing:
    Onset
    Precipitating factors
    Frequency
    Pattern
    How relieved or improved
- Impact of alteration on total well-being and life-style
- Vision:

Use of eyeglasses and date of last prescription
Date of last ophthalmologic examination
Inspection of eyes
Ability to read Snellen chart, newsprint, and large print and
to differentiate items on food tray
Visual field (Box 8-4)
- Hearing:
Use of hearing aid, when and how obtained
Date of last audiometric examination
Inspection of ears: swelling, redness, drainage, cerumen, foreign matter
Ability to hear normal conversation, watch ticking, whisper, consonants
Weber test: vibrating tuning fork is placed on forehead; if sensorineural loss is present, client will hear tone in unimpaired ear; if conductive loss is present, client will hear tone better in impaired ear; with equal bilateral deafness or normal hearing, tones will be heard equally in both ears
Rinne test: vibrating tuning fork is placed on mastoid process (bony prominence behind ear) and then removed and

---

BOX 8-4   Assessing Visual Field

This test provides a gross estimation of visual field and can be helpful in understanding adjustments that may have to be made in care. An ophthalmologist can test visual field with a target screen to obtain the most accurate evaluation.
1. Seat client comfortably.
2. Position yourself approximately 3 feet away facing the client at eye level.
3. Point your index finger and extend your arm so that it is out of your visual field.
4. Ask the client to stare into your eyes as you stare into the client's eyes.
5. As you and the client continue to stare, slowly bring your finger into the visual field.
6. Ask the client to inform you when he or she first can see your finger.
7. Note when client sees finger compared to when you do.
8. Repeat at various points along a 360-degree area of the visual field.
9. Record deficits in patient's chart so that care givers can plan accordingly.
(Sample entry: Extremely limited peripheral vision in left field. Intervention: Position bed so that right side faces door; keep bedside stand on right side.)

held alongside ear; if a conductive loss is present, tone will be heard louder on mastoid process; if a sensorineural loss is present or hearing is normal, tone will be louder alongside the ear; if a combined conductive and sensorineural loss is present, the tone will be heard equally at both locations
- Ability to differentiate different tactile stimuli (cold-hot, sharp-dull)
- Ability to identify common scents (vinegar, coffee, perfume)
- Ability to taste various substances (lemon, salt, sugar)
- Review of environment for contributory factors
- Medications used

Goals
- Client receives and interprets sensory stimuli accurately.
- Client is free from injury related to sensory deficits.
- Client obtains and utilizes eyeglasses or hearing aid.

Nursing Interventions
- Refer for ophthalmologic, audiometric, physical examinations as appropriate.
- Remove or minimize cause:
    Control noise.
    Adjust lighting.
    Encourage use of eyeglasses, hearing aids.
    Correct sensory deprivation or overload.
    Promote physical health (stabilization of vital signs, restoration of fluid and electrolyte balance).
    Consult with physician regarding medication change.
- Provide adequate sensory stimulation:
    Determine appropriate and desired level for individual.
    Keep client oriented with use of clocks, calendars, windows to see daylight and darkness.
    Use different fabrics, colors, fragrances in environment.
    Flavor foods (use artificial sweeteners and salt substitutes if restrictions are needed).
    Offer music, art therapy.
- Explain actions, clarify misconceptions.
- Protect client from injury:
    Limit temperature of hot water.
    Color-code faucet handles.
    Keep stairways well lighted.

Label liquids and other substances with large print; do not store noningestible substances near ingestible ones.

Elicit aid from roommate or family member to observe for hazards.

For hearing deficits:

- Remove cerumen accumulation, if present; soften wax with cerumenolytic agent and then irrigate with body temperature water under low pressure; avoid using cotton-tipped applicators, because they can push cerumen further into canal and cause an impaction.

- Communicate in a manner that maximizes the client's strengths:

  Reduce environmental noise and distractions.

  Face directly, and attract client's attention before beginning to speak.

  Speak slowly and distinctly.

  Use a loud but low-pitched voice: raising the voice in a yelling manner will raise the high-frequency sounds even higher and cause the client to hear less of the intended speech.

  Supplement words with exaggerated facial movements and body language.

  Give the client the opportunity to ask for clarification or repetition.

- Promote optimum communication at night or in darkened room:

  Use a night-light.

  Have ample light shining on you so that client can easily detect your presence and not be startled.

  Touch the client to gain attention.

  Use a flashlight to light your face and facilitate lip reading.

  Avoid interrupting other persons who may be sleeping in the same room by using a stethoscope to amplify speech; place the earpieces in the client's ear and talk into the bell-diaphragm portion; explain procedure to the client beforehand.

- Write important instructions and information to ensure client's understanding.

- Consult with an occupational therapist about recommendations for assistive devices (e.g., speaking tube, telephone with special amplifier, light signals rather than sound alarms).

- Ensure client is not avoided or socially isolated.

- Counsel client about hearing aid use (Figure 8-3):

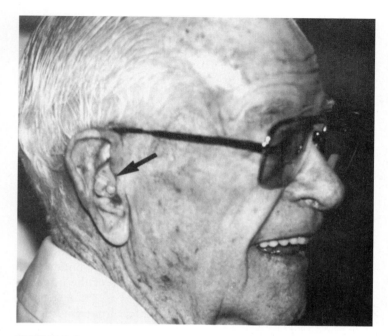

FIGURE 8-3 Hearing aids come in a variety of styles. (From Castillo HM: *The nurse assistant in long-term care: a rehabilitative approach,* St Louis, 1992, Mosby.)

Hearing aids do not benefit all persons in similar ways. Environmental sounds are amplified along with speech, causing some persons to have difficulty with adjustment. Instruct on proper care and use (Box 8-5).

For vision deficits:

• Always identify yourself when approaching client.
• Help strangers recognize client's visual deficit by providing client with a white cane or placing a sign on the bedroom door.
• Make a special effort to keep the client oriented:

Read newspapers and books to the client; read mail if client desires and approves.

Describe colors and layout of surroundings.

Have a radio available; use clocks that chime.

• Assist the client with mobility and transfers:

Have client hold your arm above elbow rather than you holding client; walk naturally.

Warn client when approaching stairs or curbs; describe depth and number.

BOX 8-5   Hearing Aids

COMPONENTS
Microphone: converts sounds into electric energy
Amplifier: increases energy
Receiver: converts energy back into sound waves
Volume control
On/off switch

STYLES
Behind the ear: limited amplification
In the ear: entire unit worn in the ear; limited amplification
Eyeglass attached: unit built in the frame of the eyeglass; limited amplification
Body aided: amplifier housed in a case worn on body; offers most amplification
  of all

NURSING CARE
- Encourage client to obtain hearing aid from a reputable dealer after a full
  audiometric examination has been done.
- Ensure that batteries are functioning before the aid is applied; it is recom-
  mended that batteries be changed weekly.
- Identify common hearing aid problems
  Whistling sound: bad connection between earpiece and amplifier; exces-
    sively high volume
  Insufficient amplification: volume set too low; weak or dead battery; block-
    age from cerumen; disconnected tubing or wiring
  Periodic loss of amplification: loose connection; poor battery contact; dirt in
    switch; cracked case
- Clean device weekly to remove cerumen and dirt
  Rotate a pipe cleaner in the opening of the earmold to remove material
  Wash earmold in warm soapy water
  Thoroughly dry
  Do not use alcohol or alcohol-based substances for cleaning
- Turn off when not in use.
- Keep away from excessive heat or cold.
- Recognize that adjustment to a hearing aid is difficult and may take time, and
  reassure the client that this is not unusual.

When seating client describe where seat is; place client's
  hand on back of seat for orientation.
- Ensure safety of environment:
    Keep doors completely open or closed.
    Remove cords, furniture, buckets, and other obstacles from
      client's path.
    Keep bed cranks in and slippers out of way.

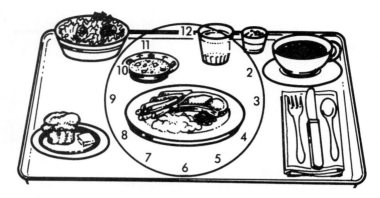

FIGURE 8-4 The concept of a clock helps a person with visual impairment to locate foods on the plate. For example, the chops are at 2 o'clock and the roll and butter are on a small plate at 8 o'clock. (From Hoeman S: *Rehabilitation/restorative care in the community,* St Louis, 1990, Mosby.)

- Place client's belongings and items on food tray in same location at all times to facilitate independent functioning. (Figure 8-4).
- Explore with occupational therapist or local service agencies the use of assistive devices (e.g., large-print or Braille books, games, and telephone dials; talking books); American Foundation for the Blind (15 W. 16th St., New York, NY 10011) can supply a catalog with hundreds of useful items.
- Support client's independence and involvement in social and life activities.

Evaluation
- Client expresses satisfaction with level of sensory input.
- Client is oriented to environment.
- Client is free from injury.
- Client uses eyeglasses or hearing aid appropriately.

Possible Related Nursing Diagnoses
Anxiety
Disturbance in self-concept
High risk for injury
Impaired social interaction
Impaired verbal communication
Social isolation

**Selected Health Problems Associated with
SENSORY-PERCEPTUAL ALTERATION:
Cataract**

GENERAL INFORMATION

A cataract is a slowly developing opacity of the lens or its capsule. Everyone develops some degree of lens opacity with age; therefore most elderly persons have some cataract formation that can cause visual impairments ranging from a sensitivity to glare to blindness.

CAUSATIVE/CONTRIBUTING FACTORS

Aging process (senile cataract)
Congenital
Eye trauma or disease
Exposure to ultraviolet B

CLINICAL MANIFESTATIONS

Gray or white opacity over pupil
Blurred vision
Increased sensitivity to glare
Progressive loss of vision

ADDITIONAL NURSING INTERVENTIONS
TO INCORPORATE INTO GENERIC CARE PLAN

- Inspect eye for gray or white opacity.
- Review history for onset and progression of visual problems, diseases present, exposure to sunlight, and trauma to eye.
- Arrange for ophthalmologic examination.
- Reduce glare with sunglasses and translucent coverings on windows to filter sunlight; use soft lights to diffuse lighting.
- Place objects within visual field.
- Monitor eye health by watching the progress of the cataract and status of the unaffected eye.
- Prepare client for surgical removal of lens:
    Early removal is recommended.
    Explain operative procedure and postoperative routines.
    Orient client to position of items in room.

Emphasize the importance of limiting intraocular pressure (e.g., avoid coughing, sneezing, bending).

Instruct client about or apply mydriatics (eye drops to dilate) and antibiotic ophthalmic ointments as prescribed.

- Give postoperative care:

Focus on client's comfort.

Observe for signs of complications (sudden eye pain, changes in vital signs).

Consult physician about proper care of soft contact or permanent intraocular implant lens.

Prepare client for need for follow-up examinations and adjustments of eyeglass prescription.

Encourage independence as soon as possible.

Glaucoma

GENERAL INFORMATION

Glaucoma is a rise of pressure within the eyeball caused by increased production and/or decreased outflow of aqueous humor. It is the second leading cause of blindness in the elderly. Glaucoma can be rapid in onset (closed-angle) or gradual (open-angle), which is the most common type.

CAUSATIVE/CONTRIBUTING FACTORS

Iritis
Allergy
Endocrine imbalance
Familial tendency

CLINICAL MANIFESTATIONS

Chronic (open-angle) glaucoma (most common type)
Gradual, subtle progression
Eyes feel tired
Gradually increasing impairment of peripheral vision
Halo around lights
Headaches (particularly in morning)
Acute (closed-angle) glaucoma

Rapid onset
Severe eye pain
Nausea, vomiting
Halo around lights
Dilated pupils
Blurred vision that can progress rapidly to blindness if
untreated

ADDITIONAL NURSING INTERVENTIONS
TO INCORPORATE INTO GENERIC CARE PLAN

- Obtain history of symptoms and evaluate visual field (see Box
  8-4).
- Arrange for ophthalmologic examination with tonometry (a
  simple test for measuring intraocular pressure).
- Encourage regular glaucoma screening in all elderly persons.
- Teach client to avoid situations that increase intraocular pressure:
      Coughing, sneezing, aggressive nose blowing
      Strenuous exercise
      Constipation, straining during defecation
      Emotional stress
- Assess extent of visual deficits and assist client with activities of
  daily living as needed.
- Counsel client to use eyes in moderation and prevent overuse
  or strain.
- Protect client from administration of drugs that could increase
  intraocular pressure (e.g., stimulants, blood pressure elevators,
  cold and allergy medications). Advise client against self-medi-
  cation with over-the-counter drugs without consulting with
  health professional.
- Advise client to inform care givers of presence of glaucoma preoperatively and when new medications are prescribed or administered.
- Encourage client to wear a bracelet or other identifying tag that
  will inform others of the presence of glaucoma if client is
  unable.
- Ensure regular evaluation by an ophthalmologist to monitor
  intraocular pressure and adjust treatment as necessary.
- Administer and instruct client to administer medications:
      Parasympathomimetics (miotics)
      Sympathomimetics

Carbonic anhydrase inhibitors
Hyperosmotic agents
- Prepare client for surgery as indicated:
  Corneal trephine
  Iridencleisis
  Sclerectomy
  Cyclocryotherapy

 Generic Care Plan:
PAIN

GENERAL INFORMATION

Pain is a state in which the individual experiences an uncomfortable sensation in response to a noxious stimulus. *Acute pain* is time limited and can be relieved (e.g., toothache, postoperative, myocardial infarction). *Chronic pain* has no predictable time limitations, and only limited relief is obtained by conventional analgesics (e.g., arthritis, shingles, phantom limb, migraine, terminal cancer). In the elderly, pain often presents itself in an altered manner, being referred to another area from its origin (e.g., gallbladder disorders can cause pain in the shoulder area) or bearing no relationship to the severity of the problem (e.g., a myocardial infarction can cause only a fluttering sensation in the chest).

CAUSATIVE/CONTRIBUTING FACTORS

Improper positioning
Restrictive clothing
High noise level
Uncomfortable temperature
Actual or impending tissue damage
Trauma
Disease process
Surgery, procedure

CLINICAL MANIFESTATIONS

Complaints of pain, discomfort, nausea
Stabbing, aching, throbbing sensations

Diaphoresis, pallor
Requests for pain medication
Increased vital signs
Crying, grimacing
Restlessness, irritability
Altered mood or behavior (confusion, depression, anxiety, irritability)
Guarded behavior

NURSING PROCESS

Assessment Considerations
- Individual pain pattern, type of pain, pain threshold
- Precipitating factors
- Frequency, duration, and intensity of pain
- Alleviating factors
- Ethnic, religious, or sexual influences on the expression of pain
- Impact on daily life (e.g., food intake, mobility, social activities)

Goals
- Client has source of pain alleviated.
- Client expresses relief from or decrease in pain.
- Client learns effective, safe measures to control pain.

Nursing Interventions
- Assist with diagnosis and treatment of underlying cause.
- Monitor pain; ask client to rate pain on scale of 0 to 10 (0 = no pain, 10 = most severe pain).
- Ensure maximum comfort by good positioning, physical support, and clean, wrinkle-free linens.
- Control environmental stimuli; alter the room temperature, provide warm or cool clothing as indicated, reduce noise level and external stimuli if contributing to pain perception.
- Gently touch client (e.g., rub brow, massage, give back rub, hold hand) to promote relaxation and comfort; use relaxation techniques, guided imagery, biofeedback, hypnosis.
- Allow client to express feelings of anger, powerlessness, anxiety.
- Be alert to newly developed symptoms or multiple complaints (e.g., knee and ankle pain may be attributed to previously diagnosed arthritis but really arises from new vascular problem).
- Review client's own pain-relief regiment to facilitate treatment by identifying successful practices and revealing potential prob-

lems (e.g., inappropriate medication use, dangerous or ineffective "fad" cures).
- Minimize impact of pain on total health by preserving energy, providing adequate nutrition, encouraging eating and activity.
- Monitor intake and output, sleep-rest pattern, activities, self-care capacity.
- Perform range-of-motion exercises if mobility is reduced.
- Maintain independence, normality, and individuality.
- Assess need for medication and evaluate effectiveness (Table 8-1):

    Begin with weakest form of analgesics; increase gradually.
    Remember that nonnarcotics will be less sedating; will have fewer, less severe side effects; and are nonaddictive.
    Administer analgesics regularly to maintain constant blood levels, maximize relief.
    Administer narcotic analgesics with caution in the elderly; there can be serious side effects, psychologic and physiologic dependency.
    Give nonnarcotic analgesics with narcotics to reduce required dosage of narcotic.
    Monitor vital signs carefully (particularly respirations) in all persons receiving narcotics.

- Support other pain relief interventions, such as surgery, chemical rhizotomy, transcutaneous electrical nerve stimulation (TENS).

Evaluation
- Client verbalizes comfort, absence or decrease of pain.
- Client participates in activities of daily living to maximum degree possible.

Possible Related Nursing Diagnoses
Activity intolerance
Altered nutrition: less than body requirements
Anxiety
Impaired social interactions
Powerlessness
Self-care deficit
Sleep pattern disturbance

TABLE 8-1   Analgesics

Examples	Common side effects	Nursing implications
NONNARCOTICS		
Acetaminophen	Irritating to gastric	Be alert to signs of
Aspirin	mucosa	infection (can mask
	Prolonged bleeding time,	associated fever)
	gastrointestinal	Give with food or milk
	bleeding (aspirin)	to reduce risk of
	Salicylate toxicity:	gastric bleeding/
	tinnitus, hearing loss,	irritation; follow
	dizziness, vomiting,	with a full glass of
	burning in mouth,	water; do not give
	throat, sweating, fever,	aspirin with fruit
	confusion, convulsions,	juice
	coma	Observe for increased
		bleeding tendency
		(bruising, bleeding
		gums)
		Can alter test
		readings for
		glycosuria
NARCOTICS		
Codeine	Drowsiness, dizziness	Protect from
Morphine	Skin rash, itching	accidents
	Nausea, vomiting	
Meperidine	Hypotension, bradycardia	Reduce dosage if
	Constipation	recommended
	Dependence	
	Exaggeration of existing	
	mental impairment	
	Severe depressant	
	reaction in the elderly	
	Interference with	
	urination	
Brompton's mixture		Used primarily in
(combination of		terminal illness
methadone, ethyl		Administered orally
alcohol, cocaine,		(every four hours);
hydrochloride syrup)		effective within 30
		minutes

Continued

TABLE 8-1   Analgesics—cont'd

INTERACTIONS

Nonnarcotics

Increase effect of cortisone-like drugs, oral anticoagulants, oral antidiabetics, penicillins, furosemide, para-aminosalicylic acid (PAS) (greater risk of aspirin toxicity).

Decrease effect of probenecid, spironolactone, sulfinpyrazone.

Effects increased by large doses of vitamin C.

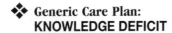Effects decreased by antacids, phenobarbital, propranolol, reserpine.

Narcotics

Increase effect of antidepressants, other analgesics, sedatives, tranquilizers.

Effects increased by antidepressants, phenothiazines, nitrates (meperidine).

Effects decreased by eye drops prescribed for glaucoma (meperidine).

❖ **Generic Care Plan:**
KNOWLEDGE DEFICIT

GENERAL INFORMATION

Knowledge deficit is a state in which the individual experiences a deficiency in cognitive knowledge or psychomotor skills that alters or threatens to alter health maintenance.

CAUSATIVE/CONTRIBUTING FACTORS

Sensory deficit
      Visual impairment
      Poor hearing
Ineffective coping
      Denial
      Anxiety
Alzheimer's disease, other cognitive deficits
New illness or treatment
Cultural practices, language differences
Impaired learning ability
Ineffective teaching

CLINICAL MANIFESTATIONS

Expresses lack of knowledge or inaccurate knowledge

Noncompliance with health practices or medical treatment

Appears to be anxious or depressed related to misinformation or lack of information

NURSING PROCESS

Assessment Considerations

- Clarify learning needs with client
- Evaluate learning ability
  - Intellectual capacity (memory, attention span, communication skills, problem-solving capability)
  - Learning and skills (literacy, calculation ability, knowledge base, educational achievements)
  - Psychomotor skills (motor dexterity, balance, equilibrium, sensation, mobility)
  - Emotional capacity (acceptance of illness or disability, control, self-image, motivation, readiness to learn)
  - Physical capacity (energy levels, vision, hearing, speech, general health)
- Current knowledge level
  - Previous experience
  - Independent learning
  - Beliefs

Goals

- Client participates in learning activities.
- Client can repeat or demonstrate knowledge and skills for health management.

Nursing Interventions

- Prepare client for educational experience by explaining the purpose of the instruction and providing an overview of what will be taught.
- Try to schedule a specific time in advance so that client can prepare self, invite family members, avoid scheduling other activities.
- Provide an environment conducive to learning that is quiet, clean, private, relaxing, and odor free.
- Give instruction time to the client exclusively with no interruptions.

- Select a teaching method appropriate to the client's abilities and needs:

  > A highly educated person may benefit from reading materials and follow-up discussion.

  > An illiterate person may require a diagrammed flip chart presentation followed by an audiotape or videotape left at the bedside for repeated review.

  > Provide opportunity for practice of skills; literature may be sufficient to teach a diabetic diet, but people require hands-on practice with needle and syringe to gain skills for insulin administration.

- Use a variety of methods to present the content: lecture, flip charts, diagrams, pamphlets, books, demonstrations, audiovisual media, group sessions, discussions with other clients who have similar condition.
- Determine priorities (e.g., of the many different facts taught to newly diagnosed diabetics, how to administer insulin and eat properly are of more immediate concern than recognizing possible complications).
- Close with a summary of content and an opportunity for the client to ask questions.
- Leave written material describing the content presented for the client's and family's later review; write a summary in the style and on the level that the client understands.
- Evaluate the effectiveness of the education:

  > Obtain feedback from client and family.

  > Observe the client for use of new knowledge and skills.

  > Ask questions informally, at a later time, to confirm understanding.

- Document information taught, when, who was involved, and effectiveness.
- Know that local, public, and college libraries, health departments, professional organizations, information and referral services, and special interest groups can provide excellent supplementary and educational materials.

Evaluation

- Client verbalizes accurate knowledge pertaining to condition and related care.
- Client demonstrates behaviors and skills consistent with desired health practices.
- Client complies with treatment plan.

Possible Related Nursing Diagnoses
Altered health maintenance
Anxiety
Noncompliance
Potential for injury
Powerlessness

RECOMMENDED READINGS

Abraham AL, Neundorfer MM: Alzheimer's: a decade of progress, a future of nursing challenges, *Geriatr Nurs* 11(3):116, 1990.
Bixen CE: Aging and mental health care, *J Gerontol Nurs* 14(11):11, 1988.
Brock CD, Simpson WM: Dementia, depression or grief? The differential diagnosis, *Geriatrics* 45(10):37, 1990.
Duffy LM, Hepburn K, Christensen R, Brugge-Wiger P: A research agenda in care for patients with Alzheimer's disease, *Image J Nurs Scholarship* 21:254, 1989.
Ebersole P: *Caring for the psychogeriatric client,* New York, 1989, Springer-Verlag.
Fidler GS, Bristow B: *Recapturing competence: a system's change for geropsychiatric care,* New York, 1992, Springer.
Foreman MD: Complexities of acute confusion, *Geriatr Nurs* 11(3):136, 1990.
Gomez G, Gomez EA: Dementia or delirium? *Geriatr Nurs* 10(3):141, 1989.
Hogstel MO, editor: *Geropsychiatric nursing,* St Louis, 1990, Mosby.
Kupfer C: Ophthalmologic disorders. In Abrams WB, Berkow R, editors: *The Merck manual of geriatrics,* Rahway, NJ, 1990, Merck Sharp and Dohme Research Laboratories.

Self-Perception, Coping, and Stress Tolerance

Today's older population has confronted challenges and obstacles unknown to younger generations, such as world wars, the Great Depression, and epidemics. They also have faced a profoundly rapid rate of change that has required adaptation to new technologies, behaviors, and ways of thinking. The fact that most elderly have survived and adjusted to these situations is a credit to their strength and coping capacity. However, old age brings new stresses—retirement, deaths, illness, role changes—at a time when physical and emotional reserves are declining. Effective management of these stresses is crucial to prevent additional problems.

Under normal circumstances people usually have a fairly realistic image of themselves. They understand their significance, capabilities, and limitations. However, under stress and other circumstances, individuals may lose their perspective and develop altered perceptions of themselves and their world.

Distortions in perception occur when one's anxiety escalates from a moderate to a severe level. Narrowed perception and an inability to take in new information are common manifestations of high anxiety. The individual has difficulty hearing, learning, or remembering information.

Many of the realities of old age make the elderly vulnerable to self-perception problems. Older adults suffer numerous losses, have less ability to protect themselves, and are confronted with many subtle messages about their misfit in a youth-oriented society. Depression may result, creating negative and distorted perceptions about self-worth, abilities to succeed, and meaninglessness of life. It is little wonder that many elderly begin to feel vulnerable and view themselves negatively.

Coping with chronic illness is a predicament that many elderly people manage on an ongoing basis. Most older persons suffer from at least one chronic disease, with several chronic illnesses that are managed simultaneously being more common. Life-style and normal activities may need to be altered to meet care needs and illness-imposed limitations. Self-concept and role identity may be threatened. Financial burdens may ensue from the cost of illness management and reduced employment. The shift in roles and responsibilities increases the client's dependency on other family members. Constraints are placed on social activity if the client's function is limited. Overwhelmed by physical, emotional, and financial burdens, physical and psychosocial health of the entire family unit may slowly erode.

The awareness of a need to adapt to a new life-style and awareness of lifelong, perhaps progressive, illness often lead to depression. Periodic episodes are common and characterized by lack of interest in self-care, withdrawal, or suicidal comments or behaviors. The inability to face the profound reality of chronic disease can cause the client to deny the existence of the disease. This denial can occur after the client has seemed to accept the disease.

Some people react with manipulation to ensure needs are fulfilled. They need to seek attention or exercise control during times of loss. Manipulation is frequently characterized by increased dependency, involving a series of requests and instilling guilt in others. Hostility can be an expression of the bitterness at being a victim of a serious illness. Anger is often displaced on close relations or companions (e.g., spouse or care givers). Regression can occur if the illness becomes too overwhelming to manage psychologically or physically; this is demonstrated by clients relinquishing responsibility for self-care or retreating to a lesser level of functioning.

The realities that accompany aging can be overwhelming and depressing when viewed in isolation. Older adults are challenged to put these realities into perspective by viewing them in light of their entire lives. By reflecting on the lives they have lived, recognizing achievements, and identifying satisfactions, the elderly are better able to find pleasure in their current lives and cope with some of the harsh realities of the present. The process of coming to terms and deriving satisfaction with the life one has lived is an important developmental task in late life. Reminiscence is a means to facilitate this process. Ego integrity and a positive self-concept are derived from feeling positive about one's life; despair, bitterness, and depression can result from disappointment and regrets with one's life.

❖ **Generic Care Plan:**
DISTURBANCE IN SELF-CONCEPT

GENERAL INFORMATION

Disturbance in self-concept is the state in which the individual experiences or is at risk of experiencing negative feelings about himself or herself. It may be triggered by a change in body image, self-esteem, role performance, or personal identity. The physical, emotional, and social losses experienced with age play a significant role in altering the elderly's self-concept.

CAUSATIVE/CONTRIBUTING FACTORS

Change or loss of role (retirement, widowhood)
Change in body appearance or function
Dependency

CLINICAL MANIFESTATIONS

Change in appearance or function
Anger
Withdrawal
Grief, depression
Denial of problem
Self-destructive actions
New or increased dependency
Preoccupation with change or loss
Not taking responsibility for self-care
Change in life-style, role

NURSING PROCESS

Assessment Considerations
- Presence of underlying cause
- Mental status
- Impact of change on activities, roles, relationships, self-esteem
- Assistive devices or efforts that have been tried and their success
- Signs of grieving, withdrawal, denial, disturbed body image, anxiety, behavioral disorganization
- Social function

Goals
- Client demonstrates positive self-image.
- Client expresses satisfaction with life-style and activities.

Nursing Interventions
- Assist in regaining maximum function and acceptable appearance (e.g., support, rehabilitative program, use of prosthetic devices).
- Encourage social interactions with significant others; have frequent contact.
- Discuss new roles with client and encourage a process of self-discovery in establishing an altered life-style.
- Recognize accomplishments and give sincere praise.
- Provide opportunities for feelings to be expressed.
- Discuss the meaning the loss or change has for the client.
- Set limits on maladaptive behaviors and identify positive behaviors that will develop adaptive coping.
- Encourage client to make decisions and follow through on plans.
- Refer to support groups, counseling, physical therapy, or occupational therapy as necessary.
- Allow time for the grieving process and inform client of the need to grieve for loss (see discussion of grief).
- Encourage client to reminisce about the past in order to gain a perspective on life (Box 9-1).
- Provide time and encouragement for clients to discuss their lives.
- Explore client's expressed disappointments and frustrations with life or self without making judgments (e.g., rather than respond to the client's remark about feeling he or she made a mess of life with the statement "No, you didn't . . . now don't

BOX 9-1   Reminiscence

Reminiscence is a therapeutic review of one's past life to:
- Resolve current conflicts
- Illuminate the individual's past
- Organize and understand significance of past events
- Cope with the present and future
- Maximize use of long-term memory when short-term memory is poor
- Offer a comfortable mechanism for expressing self more comfortably
- Maintain identity and self-esteem

Use reminiscence to assess:
- Individual accomplishments, needs
- Self-esteem
- Cognitive function
- Emotional stability
- Unresolved conflicts
- Coping ability
- Expectations for the future

GROUP PROCESS

Use questions to initiate and guide reminiscence. Strategies could include:
- Listening actively and with interest to discussions of clients' lives
- Helping clients compile poems, oral histories, or scrapbooks of their lives
- Asking clients to share information about their past. Questions could include "What was it like to leave Europe and come to America?" "How did you celebrate holidays as a child?" "What were your parents and grandparents like?" "Did you have any pets when you were young?" "How did you spend your time as a teenager?" "What was the factory like when you started working there?"
- Playing old songs and showing old photos, newspapers or magazines, and asking what was happening in the client's life at that time
- Structuring intergenerational activities in which the old can share their past with the young
- Respecting clients' privacy so that periods of silent reminiscing are not disturbed
- Asking clients to talk about a specific event or time (e.g., "Tell me how it was to be a girl in Germany." "What was your first job like?" "What was the city like when you were a teenager?")
- Using questions to help clients explore emotional responses to past events (e.g., "How did you feel when your town was invaded during the war?" "How difficult was it for you as a young widow?" "Were you disappointed at having to quit school?")
- Gently redirecting the conversation if clients' responses are repetitious or aimless (e.g., "you mentioned that before . . . did that event have a special meaning for you?" "Let's get back to how you began your career." "How

BOX 9-1   Reminiscence—cont'd

do you feel about the problems you describe between yourself and your family?")
- Listening to clients' responses; this is the most important nursing function in reminiscence
- Informing clients of time constraints and enforcing them; if appropriate, ask clients to summarize or identify the lesson/theme of the conversation

talk like that," use reflection and open-ended questions to help the client express and explore issues).
- Help clients learn new skills and find new roles.
- Assist clients to find pleasure and meaning in life, regardless of level of function (e.g., doing for others, maintaining religious practices, developing a family history book or other legacy for future generations).

Evaluation
- Client develops new roles and functions to replace lost ones.
- Client expresses satisfaction with life lived.
- Client accepts altered appearance, function, and roles.

Possible Related Nursing Diagnoses
Altered family processes
Anxiety
Impaired physical mobility
Ineffective individual coping
Powerlessness
Sensory-perceptual alteration
Sexual dysfunction

 Selected Health Problems Associated with DISTURBANCE IN SELF-CONCEPT
Depression

GENERAL INFORMATION

Depression is a feeling of extreme sadness, self-depreciation, and lack of interest in activities of daily living. It differs from grief, which has realistic and proportionate feelings related to a real loss.

Depression is thought to affect as many as 65% of the elderly, with the highest prevalence among persons with physical illness. Some degree of depression exists in an estimated 50% to 80% of all institutionalized persons.

Dementia and depression can be confused with each other. Depression can occur in persons who are in early stages of dementia because of their awareness of the cognitive changes they are experiencing; this realization causes the risk of suicide to be a major consideration in the care of early dementia victims. On the other hand, depressed persons may appear demented because of inattention to self-care activities, dull affect, and cognitive dysfunction secondary to inadequate nutrition and sleep disorders. The false impression of dementia in depressed individuals is known as pseudodementia. The relationship and potential for misdiagnosis that can occur between depression and dementia necessitate astute assessment when signs of each disorder are evident.

CAUSATIVE/CONTRIBUTING FACTORS

Reduced levels of norepinephrine, serotonin, or their metabolites (catecholamine theory)
Poor physical health, which weakens emotional coping capacity
Medications (particularly phenothiazides, sedatives, reserpine)
Low self-esteem, guilt
Anger turned inward
Loss of role or responsibility, feeling worthless
Dependency, powerlessness
Unresolved grief
Losses: loved one, pet, home, income

CLINICAL MANIFESTATIONS

General lack of interest in life
Emotional distress
Sadness, pessimism
Helplessness, hopelessness
Apathy, emptiness
Guilt, anxiety
Listlessness, fatigue
Psychomotor slowing
Anorexia, weight loss

Constipation
Sleep disturbances
Loss of libido
Impaired cognition (secondary to poor nutrition, sleep disorder)

ADDITIONAL NURSING INTERVENTIONS
TO INCORPORATE INTO GENERIC CARE PLAN

- Review client's recent history for a precipitating event or circumstance (death, retirement, relocation, additional financial burden, new medication).
- Evaluate symptoms carefully, because they may mimic those of dementia; note any indications of dementia (decline in intellect, personality).
- Offer grief counseling, refer to widow(er)s' group for support if appropriate.
- Suggest new activities or volunteer work to build self-esteem.
- Display positive attitude toward progress and eventual outcome.
- Assist in forming new goals and providing opportunities for success.
- Consult a professional if psychotherapy seems indicated; although less effective for the elderly, this therapy can prove helpful.
- Be alert to and address secondary physical problems such as malnutrition, poor hygiene, constipation, and fatigue.
- Take hints of suicide seriously; the risk is very real; know that attempts may be very subtle (e.g., omitting needed medication, starvation).
- Exercise aggressive observation and supervision if client has suicidal ideation (see discussion of suicide, p. 293).
- Administer antidepressant medications as ordered; monitor carefully; be aware of side effects of antidepressants and evaluate effectiveness of regimen (Table 9-1).
- Explain to client that antidepressant medication can take 4 to 6 weeks before therapeutic effects are experienced.
- Be aware that frequent dosage adjustments may be necessary to achieve maximum benefits from drug therapy and the initial dosage for an older person is usually one third to one half the normal adult dosage.
- Instruct the client to continue taking antidepressant medication for several months after improvement is noted.

TABLE 9-1   **Antidepressant Drugs**

Examples	Side effects	Nursing implications

Tricyclics
  Amitriptyline
  Desipramine
  Doxepin
  Imipramine
  Nortriptyline
  Protriptyline
  Tranylcypromine
	Dry mouth, diaphoresis,
	cardiac changes, urinary
	retention
		Offer hard candies, good
		oral hygiene, fluids.
		Observe for dehydration,
		offer fluids, keep skin
		clean and dry.
		Obtain baseline and
		periodic ECG.
		Monitor vital signs.
		Monitor intake and output.

Trazodone
  hydrochloride
  Desyrel
	Increased or decreased
	appetite, red eyes, dry
	mouth, blurred vision,
	constipation
		Administer with food or
		meals.

MAO inhibitors*
  Isocarboxazid
  Phenelzine
    sulfate
  Tranylcypromine
    sulfate
  Pargyline
	Indigestion, constipation
	Toxic symptoms when taken
	with foods high in tyramine
	Hypotension, drowsiness
	Blurred vision,
	photosensitivity
	Fluctuation of blood glucose
	level
		Observe for drowsiness;
		administer major dose
		at bedtime to minimize
		problems associated
		with this reaction.
		Observe serum levels of
		these drugs, because
		increased levels can
		occur if administered
		with digoxin or
		phenytoin.
		Monitor vital signs.
		Advise that positions be
		changed slowly.
		Ensure adequate
		nutritional intake,
		monitor bowel
		elimination, incorporate
		foods in diet that will
		ease digestion and
		prevent constipation.
		Teach client to avoid
		foods such as alcohol,
		chocolate, avocado,
		yeast extract, pickled
		herrings, pods of broad
		beans, chicken livers,
		and processed or aged
		cheese.

TABLE 9-1 Antidepressant Drugs—cont'd

Examples	Side effects	Nursing implications
		Monitor vital signs.
		Advise that positions be changed slowly.
		Observe closely.
		Supervise activities.
		Ensure safety of environment.
		Advise to wear sunglasses and use other measures to screen sun.
		Monitor blood glucose.
		Observe for signs of hypoglycemia and hyperglycemia.

*MAO Inhibitors can have devastating effects on the aged and are not frequently prescribed.

Interactions
Increase effects of anticoagulants, atropine-like drugs, antihistamines, sedatives, tranquilizers, narcotics, levodopa.
Decrease effects of clonidine, phenytoin, guanethidine, various antihypertensives.
Effects increased by thiazide diuretics, alcohol.

Mania

GENERAL INFORMATION

Mania is a mental disorder characterized by a euphoric mood, excessive excitement, and hyperactive behaviors. Many elderly manics have rapid swings between mania and depression; however, less than 10% of all manic-depressive reactions are manic.

CAUSATIVE/CONTRIBUTING FACTORS

Affective psychosis
Meningovascular syphilis
Medication (stimulants)
Alcohol
Psychodynamics

CLINICAL MANIFESTATIONS

Elevated mood, elation
Accelerated activity, thought processes, speech
Reduced sleep
Aggressive behavior
Irritability
Delirium (in severe cases)

ADDITIONAL NURSING INTERVENTIONS
TO INCORPORATE INTO GENERIC CARE PLAN

- Minimize stimulation by:
    Restricting noise including television and radio, traffic (staff, visitors)
    Avoiding temperature extremes (maintain environmental temperature of about 75° F)
    Giving short explanations (do not try to reason or explain)
- Meet nutritional needs by providing foods that can be eaten simply and quickly; a high-calorie, high-protein diet is beneficial.
- Offer fluids frequently; monitor intake and output.
- Encourage and allow client to rest when he or she desires.
- Protect others from client and protect client from humiliating self by helping client to control bizarre behavior, sexual acting out, etc.
- Administer medications (e.g., tranquilizers, lithium) as prescribed; monitor blood levels of medications and signs of adverse reactions; be aware that the half-life of these drugs can be prolonged in the elderly and that initial dosage should be low with gradual increases if necessary.

❖ Generic Care Plan:
ANXIETY

GENERAL INFORMATION

Anxiety is a state in which the individual experiences feelings of uneasiness, apprehension, and impending doom. The autonomic nervous system is activated in response to a vague, nonspecific threat. Anxiety differs from fear in that the threat is not identifiable. It is a common psychiatric problem experienced by the elderly.

Symptoms associated with anxiety can occur on a variety of levels along a continuum, ranging from mild anxiety experienced over minor problems to panic (Figure 9-1). Also, several anxiety-related problems can exist. For instance, profound feelings of anxiety, known as *panic attacks,* can develop for no apparent reason; a fear of being in anxiety-causing situations that causes specific actions to be taken to avoid these situations can exist and is referred to as *agoraphobia;* and anxiety can result from recurrent images of past stressful events with *posttraumatic stress disorder.* A thorough assessment is essential in identifying the specific type and cause of anxiety.

CAUSATIVE/CONTRIBUTING FACTORS

Multiple losses (status, role, possessions, people)
Reduced income, increased expenses
Loneliness
Social isolation
Chronic illness, invasive procedures
Change in environment (hospitalization, relocation)
Retirement, unemployment
Medical condition causing anxiety as a symptom (e.g., hyperthyroidism, cardiac arrhythmia, pulmonary emboli)
Drugs (e.g., anticholinergics)
Delirium, hypochondriasis, dementia

CLINICAL MANIFESTATIONS

Physiologic
    Rapid pulse, chest pain, increased blood pressure
    Tremors, trembling, increased psychomotor activity
    Profuse perspiration; cold, clammy hands
    Headaches, dizziness
    Sleep disturbances
    Change in appetite (increased or decreased)
    Change in bowel elimination pattern (increased or decreased)
    Dry mouth, indigestion, nausea
    Urinary frequency

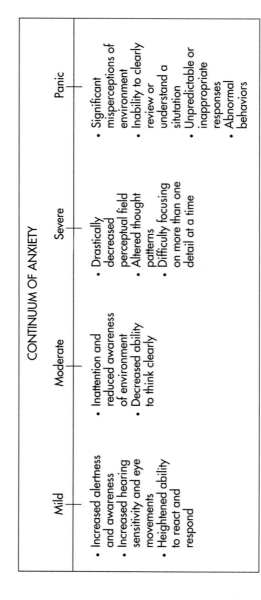

CONTINUUM OF ANXIETY

Mild	Moderate	Severe	Panic
• Increased alertness and awareness • Increased hearing sensitivity and eye movements • Heightened ability to react and respond	• Inattention and reduced awareness of environment • Decreased ability to think clearly	• Drastically decreased perceptual field • Altered thought patterns • Difficulty focusing on more than one detail at a time	• Significant misperceptions of environment • Inability to clearly review or understand a situation • Unpredictable or inappropriate responses • Abnormal behaviors

FIGURE 9-1 Continuum of anxiety. (From Eliopoulos C: Helping the resident with anxiety, *Long Term Care Educator* 5[5]:5, 1994.)

Aching muscles, tension
Sweating, hot or cold spells
Dyspnea, hyperventilation
Cognitive
Difficulty concentrating, confusion
Poor memory
Rumination, asking same question repeatedly
Orientation to past rather than present or future
Emotional
Apprehension
Helplessness
Fears or phobias
Irritability
Angry outbursts
Crying
Losing control
Criticism of self and others
Nervousness

NURSING PROCESS

Assessment Considerations
- Health status, physical condition, mental status, diagnoses
- Medications
- Recent changes or new stresses (e.g., death of pet, relocation, recently diagnosed illness, reduced income)
- Level of anxiety and client's perception of the threat represented by the situation
- Life situation of family; coping style

Goal
- Client recognizes and develops coping mechanism to reduce and manage anxiety.

Nursing Interventions
- Eliminate or correct underlying cause if possible (e.g., improve health status, obtain financial aid, help secure home, provide support system).
- Reduce environmental stimuli such as glare, bright lights, and noise, stabilize room temperature; control interruptions and traffic flow.

- Adjust care activities to limit frustration and uncertainty; establish and maintain consistent routines.
- Teach stress reduction techniques such as deep breathing, visualization, meditation.
- Explain procedures and activities to divert attention.
- Offer a warm bath, back rub, or warm milk.
- Encourage expression of feelings and help client to label feelings of anxiety and so on.
- Minimize client's responsibilities and decisions.
- Guide client in finding solutions to problems.
- Assess need for antianxiety medication and give to client as prescribed; be aware of side effects and interactions (Table 9-2).
- Be aware that antipsychotic medications are not recommended for generalized anxiety unless signs of psychoses are present.
- Ensure that lowest possible dosage (age adjusted) of medication is ordered and that drugs are withdrawn gradually to avoid ill consequences associated with physiologic and psychologic dependency that may exist.
- Review history for conditions that would contraindicate use of antianxiety drugs (e.g., acute alcohol intoxication; myasthenia

TABLE 9-2   Antianxiety Drugs

Examples	Side effects	Nursing implications
SHORT-ACTING BENZODIAZEPINES		
Alprazolam (Xanax) Lorazepam (Ativan) Oxazepam (Serax)	Drowsiness, ataxia, slurred speech, sleep disturbances, constipation, gastrointestinal upset, nausea, vomiting	Shorter-acting benzodiazepines tend to cause better response in elderly than longer-acting agents. Maintain adequate fluid and nutrient intake. Monitor nutritional status, intake and output, and bowel elimination.

TABLE 9-2 Antianxiety Drugs—cont'd

Examples	Side effects	Nursing implications
		Protect from falls and other injuries associated with side effects.
LONG-ACTING BENZODIAZEPINES		
Chlordiazepoxide hydrochloride (Librium) Clorazepate (Tranxene) Diazepam (Valium) Halazepam (Paxipam) Prazepam (Centrax)	Drowsiness, lethargy, weakness, fainting, unsteady gait, delirium, slurred speech, impaired bladder control	Advise client to change positions slowly; avoid driving, operating machinery, and engaging in any other activity that requires mental alertness. Monitor mental status; keep oriented. Toilet frequently. Protect from falls and other injuries associated with side effects.
AZAPIRONES		
Buspirone (BuSpar)	Nausea, vomiting, gastrointestinal upset, dizziness, drowsiness, headache, sleep disturbances, fatigue	Several weeks of drug therapy may be needed for clinical benefit to be realized; support client during this time. Monitor nutritional status and intake and output. Protect from falls and other injuries associated with side effects.

Interactions
Increased effects of anticonvulsants, antihypertensives, oral anticoagulants, other CNS depressants.
Effects increased by tricyclic antidepressants.
Combined with anticonvulsants, can increase seizure activity.

gravis; blood dyscrasias; acute narrow-angle glaucoma; severe pulmonary, hepatic, or renal disease).
- Prevent complications related to medication side effects, such as falls or infections.
- Refer for and support psychotherapy as appropriate.

Evaluation
- Client reports reduction in level of anxiety.
- Client develops and uses new coping mechanisms.

Possible Related Nursing Diagnoses
Disturbance in self-concept
Impaired social interactions
Ineffective individual coping
Knowledge deficit
Sleep pattern disturbance
Social isolation

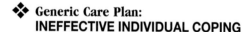

❖ **Generic Care Plan:**
   INEFFECTIVE INDIVIDUAL COPING

GENERAL INFORMATION

Ineffective individual coping is the impairment of adaptive behaviors and problem-solving abilities of a person in meeting life's demands and roles.

CAUSATIVE/CONTRIBUTING FACTORS

Situational crises
Maturational crises
Unrealistic and/or unmet expectations
Poor health habits, nutrition, or exercise
Multiple life changes and losses
Chronic illness
Inadequate support systems
Inadequate coping methods

CLINICAL MANIFESTATIONS

Destructive behavior toward self or others
High rate of frequent illness and/or accidents
Change in communication patterns
Inability to meet role expectations
Verbalization of "I can't cope"
Inability to problem solve
Excessive smoking, drinking, or drug use
Insomnia or fatigue
Irritability, worrying, anxiety, or tension
Frequent complaints of headache, gastrointestinal symptoms, aches and pains that seem unrelated to any physical problem
Denial
Manipulation
Hostility
Regression
Grief

NURSING PROCESS

Assessment Considerations

- History of contributing factors (e.g., recent change in life-style, new health problem, added responsibility, loss of significant other)
- Lifelong pattern of coping
- Functional capacity
- Risks resulting from ineffective coping, such as potential suicide, malnutrition, accidents, victimization, harm to others
- Degree of impairment
- Ability of client and family to understand current situation

Goal

- Client and/or family identifies effective strategies to manage stress.

Nursing Interventions

- Assist with diagnosis and treatment of underlying cause.
- Encourage communication with others and converse at client's level.
- Encourage expression of anxieties, fears, anger, frustration; convey to client these are normal reactions.

- Assess family health, strengths, weaknesses, and relationships to determine members' real ability to assist the client.
- Address family needs in the care plan; ensure members' ability to assist and cope with long-term client problems.
- Ensure client and care givers understand realities of disease and its management.
- Explain procedures before doing in a simple, clear manner.
- Use clocks, calendars, and pictures to keep client oriented to time and place.
- Support client in evaluating life-style and necessary changes to be made.
- Explore management alternatives with the family to derive acceptable and workable approaches.
- Aid client in gaining more effective problem-solving and stress management techniques:
  Discuss how client can recognize issues and clearly identify the consequences of various actions.
  Describe available resources to assist, such as support groups, counselors, hot lines.
- Develop goals; long-term goals give a sense of direction and outcome; short-term goals offer milestones on which to measure progress.
- Teach relaxation exercises and strategies (daily sessions of soft music with eyes closed, yoga, meditation, physical exercise).
- Prioritize care plans to ensure that the most pressing client and family needs are given maximum attention.
- Refer for psychiatric care as appropriate.

Evaluation
- Client and/or family implements effective alternatives to manage stress.
- Client and/or family identifies and utilizes coping abilities.

Possible Related Nursing Diagnoses
Anxiety
High risk for injury
Ineffective family coping
Powerlessness
Sleep pattern disturbance

❖ Selected Health Problems Associated with INEFFECTIVE INDIVIDUAL COPING Suicide

GENERAL INFORMATION

Suicide is the act of taking one's own life voluntarily and intentionally. Suicidal behaviors are self-destructive actions that can result in death.

Twenty-five percent of all suicides occur in persons over 65 years of age, with the highest rate among white males over 75 years of age. The elderly have more successful completed suicide attempts than younger age groups.

CAUSATIVE/CONTRIBUTING FACTORS

Depression and factors causing depression
    Widowhood
    Retirement without meaningful role to replace work role
    Relocation (within past 2 years)
    Poverty (primarily those who become poor in old age)
    Social isolation and loneliness
    Crises
Low impulse control
Significant losses incurred
Psychiatric problems

CLINICAL MANIFESTATIONS

Overt attempt (e.g., overdosing, shooting self, hanging)
Purposeful accidents
Omission of therapeutic measures
Self-mutilation
Depression
Vague statements about ending one's life
Alcoholism
Storing medications
Hostility
Despair or despondency
Hopelessness or helplessness
Grief

Withdrawal or isolation
Ambivalence
Inability to cope
Recent purchase of weapon

ADDITIONAL NURSING INTERVENTIONS
TO INCORPORATE INTO GENERIC CARE PLAN

- Refer for crisis intervention.
- Assess client for level of lethality and degree of risk to self.
- Identify precipitating event that was the "last straw" for the client: what happened and what is the specific meaning of the event to the individual.
- Assess the client's coping strategies and what has been done in past when these feelings surfaced.
- Assess client's level of impulse control and presence of excessive drinking or drug use.
- Identify significant others and social resources who can be notified of the client's suicidal intention.
- Review past suicide attempts, methods used, and why attempts failed.
- Explore past psychiatric history, chronic illnesses, and previous contacts with counselors or hot lines.
- Review current life-style, recent losses, and changes.
- Ask client directly: "Do you have a plan? What is it? When do you plan on carrying it out? Do you have the means to implement your plan (pills, gun, etc.)?"
- Encourage the expression of feelings of hopelessness and despair, give empathy for the situation, and reflect back to client your understanding of the dilemma.
- Realize all suicidal people are ambivalent and appeal to the part of the client who wants to live.
- Point out to the client that he or she wants to kill the emotional pain, not himself or herself, but that the two are merged in the mind.
- Remove dangerous items from the environment (e.g., razor blades, medications, guns).
- Have someone stay with the client until the crisis is over.
- Make a verbal or written contract with the client, stating he or she will call you or someone else (designate who) before a suicide attempt.

- Lend perspective about the problem; give the client another way to view the situation.
- Identify new coping mechanisms, and assist the client in developing constructive ways to manage the problem.
- Reinforce positive attributes and behaviors.
- Refer for psychiatric care and support follow-up sessions.

Alcoholism

GENERAL INFORMATION

Alcoholism is the abuse, dependency, or addiction to alcohol that threatens physical, emotional, and social health. Alcoholism in late life is more prevalent among persons who have used alcohol throughout their lives. Older persons are less able to detoxify and excrete alcohol, and therefore they are more vulnerable to its effects. Alcoholism decreases the ability to cope with age-related physical, mental, and socioeconomic changes. It can increase morbidity and mortality from many otherwise unrelated health problems. Early detection is crucial since the shorter the history of the problem the greater the chance of recovery. It is important that alcoholism be differentiated from other problems causing similar signs, such as early dementia and cerebrovascular accident. Active intervention can help prevent alcohol abuse among high-risk elderly such as lonely, depressed, widowed, and poor persons.

CAUSATIVE/CONTRIBUTING FACTORS
Loneliness or depression
Low self-esteem
Poor health
Poor coping abilities
Dependency traits
Lifelong pattern
Familial tendency

CLINICAL MANIFESTATIONS
Dependence on alcohol to relieve tension
Memory blackouts
Poor nutritional status

Disrupted personal relationships
Social isolation
Arrests for minor violations or driving offenses
While intoxicated:
     Decreased inhibitions
     Clumsiness or staggering
     Mood fluctuation
     Anger or depression
Signs of related complications
     Gastritis
     Nutritional deficiencies
     Cirrhosis
     Congestive heart failure
     Fluid and electrolyte imbalances
     Hepatitis
     Osteoporosis
     Gastrointestinal bleeding
Blood alcohol level greater than 150 mg/dl

ADDITIONAL NURSING INTERVENTIONS
TO INCORPORATE INTO GENERIC CARE PLAN

- Explore drinking history and pattern, amount, frequency, form of alcoholic beverage, precipitating factors, reactions to alcohol, behavioral changes (or lack of), and alcohol tolerance.
- Observe for withdrawal signs and be aware that a decrease in alcohol consumption can cause withdrawal reactions:
     Tremors (6 to 8 hours after last drink)
     Disorientation, hallucinations, or convulsions (10 to 30 hours after last drink)
     Delirium tremens (60 to 80 hours after last drink)
- Prevent complications during withdrawal (mortality from improperly managed withdrawal is as high as 15%) by the following:
     Administering sedatives (chlordiazepotide [Librium], diazepam [Valium], other long-lasting CNS depressants) as prescribed
     Monitoring vital signs and general status carefully; an elevated pulse rate could indicate impending delirium tremens
     Gradually withdrawing drugs once client has stabilized

Preventing and/or managing seizures by administering magnesium, keeping environment quiet and nonstimulating, maintaining hydration and good nutrition, and offering emotional support
- Assess for symptoms of possible complications (e.g., jaundice, edema, altered cognition, disorientation, memory deficits, tremors, stupor, pain, congestive heart failure).
- Maintain and improve nutritional status by providing well-balanced meals, supplements, and fluids because:

    Wernicke-Korsakoff syndrome (result of chronic alcoholism) is related to thiamine deficiencies from alcoholism.

    Magnesium deficiencies can develop from chronic alcoholism.

    Polyneuropathy occurs mainly among malnourished alcoholics.

    Gastritis and pancreatitis often occur in alcoholics.
- Administer medications as prescribed.
- Be knowledgeable of signs and symptoms related to drug interactions:

    Alcohol interacts with analgesics, antibiotics, anticoagulants, anticonvulsants, antidepressants, antihistamines, barbiturates, digitalis, diuretics, insulin, and iron preparations.

    Alcohol can cause a tolerance to barbiturates, hypnotics, sedatives, and tranquilizers.
- Help client deal with the underlying reason for drinking.
- Help family and client accept diagnosis and support client's efforts to quit.
- Refer to Alcoholics Anonymous (AA), detoxification units, Al-anon, and other community resources once the client accepts that there is a problem with alcohol.

❖ **Generic Care Plan:**
POWERLESSNESS

GENERAL INFORMATION

Powerlessness is a state in which an individual perceives a lack of personal control over certain events or situations. It occurs when one perceives that personal actions will not significantly affect an outcome. These individuals tend to have an external locus of control and believe chance, luck, or fate determines one's life events. The elderly are particularly vulnerable since they often have fewer resources, less physical strength, diminished social support, and decreased self-esteem, all of which increase vulnerability to powerlessness. In addition, psychosocial and physiologic changes inherent in the aging process often lead to an experience of powerlessness. The potential reactions to these feelings can threaten the older person's self-care capacity and quality of life.

CAUSATIVE/CONTRIBUTING FACTORS

Illness, particularly those that debilitate or increase dependency
Sensory deficits
Psychomotor limitations
Losses (status, money, support persons)
Lack of information or skill
Hospitalization or institutionalization
Loss of meaningful work or activities
Stereotyping that denotes inferiority
Life-style of helplessness

CLINICAL MANIFESTATIONS

Expressed feelings of not being in control of situation
Failure or inability to make decisions
Apathy or depression
Aggressive behavior, acting-out, anger, or resentment
Passivity
Anxiety

NURSING PROCESS

Assessment Considerations
- Underlying cause such as new situation, immobility, illness, lack of knowledge
- Decision-making ability, coping ability, ability to control life, responsibilities
- Effects of powerlessness on total function and well-being
- Locus of control (internal or external)

- Expressions of "giving up" or "no one cares" or a lack of communication
- Manipulative behavior
- Responses to treatments

Goals
- Client identifies reasons for feeling powerless.
- Client identifies and uses ways to increase sense of self-control.

Nursing Interventions
- Eliminate or correct underlying cause if possible (e.g., provide information, teach new skills, obtain assistive devices).
- Refer for and support psychotherapy.
- Allow maximum control and participation in self-care activities.
- Provide explanations, and prepare client for procedures.
- Respect client's desires and decisions.
- Demonstrate concern and caring by listening and encouraging expressions of anger, apathy, and hopelessness.
- Modify environment to increase client's control (e.g., call bell, telephone, television within easy reach).
- Assist client to set realistic goals and discuss probable outcomes and objectives to reaching desired result.
- Assist client to maintain an internal locus of control by indicating how events are often determined by one's own behavior; this focus not only gives the person a sense of power, but also inspires hope that choices are available.
- Give matter-of-fact feedback to client about manipulative behavior; offer alternative ways to get needs met.
- Assist client to identify what he or she can do for self.

Evaluation
- Client expresses reduction in feelings of powerlessness.
- Client demonstrates increased control over decisions and activities.

Possible Related Nursing Diagnoses
Disturbance in self-concept
Ineffective individual coping
Knowledge deficit
Sensory-perceptual alterations
Sleep pattern disturbance
Social isolation

RECOMMENDED READINGS

Bixen CE: Aging and mental health care, *J Gerontol Nurs* 14(11):11, 1988.

Blazer D: Depression in the elderly, *N Engl J Med* 320(3):164, 1989.

Blazer D, Bachar J, Manton K: Suicide in late life, *J Am Geriatr Soc* 36(7): 519, 1986.

Brock CD, Simpson WM: Dementia, depression or grief? The differential diagnosis, *Geriatrics* 45(10):37, 1990.

Buckwalter KC: How to unmask depression, *Geriatr Nurs* 11(4):179, 1990.

Hogstel MO, editor: *Geropsychiatric nursing,* St Louis, 1990, Mosby.

NIH Consensus Conference: Diagnosis and treatment of depression in late life, *JAMA* 268(8), 1992.

10

❖ Role Relationship

A role consists of the behaviors and expectations associated with a particular social position (e.g., spouse, parent, or employee). Roles are learned through a socialization process early in life; thus an inadequate or unrealistic socialization, or the confrontation of an unfamiliar role, can hinder the adequate fulfillment of roles, such as in the following examples:

- A man whose father abused his wife and children may be abusive with his own wife and children.
- A woman who has known the role of homemaker throughout her adult life may not understand how to meet the demands of the workplace now that she is widowed and in need of paid employment.

Over the life span, roles can change because of age (e.g., parent-child relationships), new responsibilities (e.g., remarriage), and altered status (e.g., retirement). The major factors influencing the aging person's ability to cope with role changes include the following:

- Health status
- Experience
- Financial resources
- Education
- Support systems

ROLE CHANGES

Parenthood
As children become adults and leave their parental homes parents lose the focus of many of their daily activities. If parents have not

developed other sources of activity and fulfillment they may feel a significant loss and stress from this change in parental role, referred to as the empty nest syndrome.

With increased age there is a greater likelihood that roles will be reversed. After years of being responsible for their children, parents depend on children for decision making, financial support, and other forms of assistance. This can be a difficult adjustment for both parents and their offspring.

Also there can be conflict if adult children remain living in their parents' homes, which more children are doing for longer periods of time. Parents may feel torn between a sense of obligation to their offspring and a desire to be free of daily family responsibilities.

Grandparenthood

A majority of older people are grandparents, and they meet this role with a variety of styles. Some grandparents assume an active role in the support, care, and guidance of their grandchildren, whereas others are remote, visiting only on special occasions and having minimal involvement. For most persons, the grandparent role is more satisfying than stressful; dissatisfaction may result when expectations of grandparents or grandchildren differ from the actual roles assumed.

Retirement

Retirees must adjust to the loss of the job-related sense of purpose, worth, and identity and the absence of daily structure that filled large blocks of time. The degree to which these needs are met through other means will determine the success of retirement.

It is not unusual for a person's early anticipation of retirement to be unrealistic. "Now I can play golf as much as I want." "I'll finally be able to travel all the time." Initially on retirement there is excitement as one attempts to fulfill dreams. Eventually this often gives way to boredom and unhappiness with all of the unstructured time. "I don't seem to enjoy golf as much now that I can play it whenever I want." Economic constraints also may limit one's fulfillment of dreams. "After paying my basic living expenses there isn't much left to use for travel." Retirees may need support and counseling to minimize stress and develop meaningful roles to substitute for the work role.

Widowhood

The likelihood of becoming widowed increases with each advancing year. For women, widowhood is a significant problem primarily because women enjoy a longer life expectancy than men and tend to marry men older than themselves. The major factors affecting adjustment to widowhood include cultural background, age, relationship with spouse, financial status, and support systems.

Grief usually is most intense during the first 2 months after the spouse's death, followed by 1 year of significant but less intense mourning. The widowed person's adjustment should be monitored during this time. The widowhood role solidifies approximately 2 years after the spouse's death. Widowed persons may need support and guidance in the following tasks:

- Developing an identity as a single person
- Learning to manage expenses or a household
- Adjusting to a reduced income
- Exploring new relationships
- Establishing sexual relationships
- Contemplating remarriage
- Organizing life-style

A new, lost, or changed role can be a double-edged sword. It can bring emptiness and devastation or growth and challenge. Individuals need to be viewed in relation to the world in which they interact to fully understand the many facets of their being. Each social position and function draw out different aspects, carries expectations of behavior, and impact in various ways.

Many of the losses and illnesses of late life can lead to a change in body image, identity, and responses. This can cause the elderly to view themselves negatively and interfere with their social interactions and satisfactory fulfillment of roles and responsiblities. These impairments must be eliminated or minimized to avoid additional risks to health and well-being.

Nursing staff can assist older adults in coping with losses and changes by offering maximum opportunities for choice and control, even with seemingly minor decisions, and assisting them in establishing new roles and relationships. Identifying and building on the unique capabilities and assets of older individuals, rather than focusing on losses and limitations, are important approaches to helping the elderly achieve a sense of psychosocial well-being.

❖ Generic Care Plan:
IMPAIRED SOCIAL INTERACTION; SOCIAL ISOLATION

GENERAL INFORMATION

Situations of impaired social interaction occur when there is an interference with contact with other people because of physical, emotional, or socioeconomic factors. A feeling of aloneness develops that can result in other problems and responses such as anxiety, depression, and poor nutrition.

Impaired social interaction exists when the individual has an excess or insufficient amount of social activity or suffers from a poor quality of social interaction.

CAUSATIVE/CONTRIBUTING FACTORS

Loss of relationship: death, relocation, divorce, hospitalization
Health problems, disabilities, pain, incontinence
Poor self-concept, disfigurement, obesity, feelings of worthlessness
Insufficient money to engage in leisure or social activities
Lack of transportation
Sensory losses: poor vision, inability to hear conversation
Altered mental status
Communication barriers: language differences, nonassertiveness

CLINICAL MANIFESTATIONS

Underactivity
Sleep disturbances: excessive sleep or insomnia
Appetite disturbances: overeating or anorexia
Depression
Anxiety, restlessness
Anger
Inability to concentrate or make decisions
Feelings of uselessness, abandonment
Desire for more contact, attention seeking
Expressed feeling that time is passing slowly

NURSING PROCESS

Assessment Considerations
- Recent changes in health status (e.g., weight gain or loss, fatigue)
- Possible causative/contributing factors
- Barriers to social interaction
- Life-style
- Lifelong pattern of socialization
- Impact on total health status

Goals
- Client establishes or reestablishes meaningful social contacts.
- Client maintains or develops supportive and nurturing relationships.

Nursing Interventions
- Assist with identification and management of underlying problem (e.g., obtaining assistive device, referring to social worker, supporting psychotherapy).
- Assist client with adaptation to new roles:
    Facilitate open discussion about role changes and their impact.
    Educate and counsel client about the realities of the role change.
    Link the client with resources and other persons in similar situations.
    Help the client find meaningful roles to substitute for lost ones or to learn skills associated with new roles.
    Monitor physical, emotional, and social status to ensure no negative impact results from role changes.
- Eliminate or minimize effects of causative or contributing factors:
    Introduce to new social contacts, senior groups, organizations.
    Link with resources for transportation, financial aid, telephone reassurance.
    Assist in management of medical problems.
    Obtain assistive devices to compensate for deficits.
    Mobilize family members, friends, neighbors.
    Recommend pets, house sharing, alternate living arrangements.

BOX 10-1   Remotivation

REMOTIVATION IS A GROUP PROCESS TO
- Improve grooming and interest in activities of daily living
- Increase interest in world and new activities; mental stimulation
- Increase communication and socialization; ability to discuss topics other than self or illness
- Promote self-worth and security through group membership

GROUP MEMBERS
- Must have enough cognitive function to participate in structured group activities and discussion.
- Six to 12 individuals meet at regular, prescheduled time several times per week

GROUP PROCESS
- Introduce group members and establish a warm, friendly tone.
- Conduct reality orientation by
  Reviewing current events
  Leading group discussions on such topics as flowers, foreign countries, art objects, clothing, school(s), literature
  Eliciting comments, reactions, ideas from *all* members
  Acknowledging *all* contributions
- Include an ongoing special activity (e.g., assembling a book, planting a garden, planning a trip).
- Summarize each meeting and express appreciation for members' participation.

Recommend participation in a remotivation group (Box 10-1).
- Keep in mind that a certain amount of solitude is healthy for all persons; choosing to be alone is different from the inability to have social contact (Figure 10-1).

Evaluation
- Client expresses satisfaction with level of social activity.
- Client is free from secondary problems related to poor social interaction.

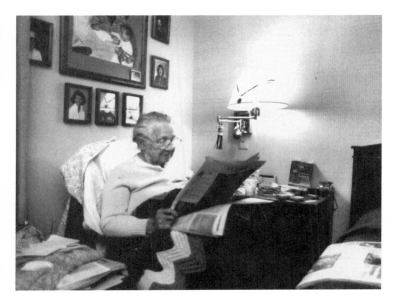

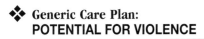

FIGURE 10-1 A certain amount of solitude is healthy for all persons.

Possible Related Nursing Diagnoses
Activity intolerance
Altered nutrition
Anxiety
Disturbance in self-concept
Fear
Impaired verbal communication
Powerlessness
Sleep pattern disturbance

❖ **Generic Care Plan:**
POTENTIAL FOR VIOLENCE

GENERAL INFORMATION

Potential for violence is a state in which the client is at risk for developing, or has demonstrated, aggressive behaviors. These behaviors can be a threat to the client (self-destructive) or others.

CAUSATIVE/CONTRIBUTING FACTORS

Toxic reactions to medications, alcohol
Dementia
Delirium
Hormonal imbalance
Paranoia
Overwhelming stress (e.g., care giving)
Fear, misperceptions
Catastrophic event
Uncontrolled anger
Being victim of violence

CLINICAL MANIFESTATIONS

Body language: clenched fists, increased motor activity, angry-looking facial expression
Overt aggressive acts: hitting, punching, kicking
Evidence of self-injury, bruises, scratches
Expressed threats and anger
Fear, anxiety, suspiciousness
Self-destructive acts

NURSING PROCESS

Assessment Considerations
- Evidence of violent acts to self and others
- History of use of violence, abuse
- Precipitating events: bad experience, new use of alcohol or drugs
- Physical examination
- Mental status evaluation

Goals
- Client gains control over behavior.
- Client is free from violent acts against self and others.
- Client learns constructive ways to express feelings.

Nursing Interventions
- Assist with identification and treatment of underlying cause.
- Discuss behavior with client; set limits and consequences of exceeding limits of acceptable behavior (e.g., will not be taken on field trip, will be placed in seclusion).

- Aid client in developing nonviolent means of expressing feelings (e.g., talking out feelings, walking, physical activity).
- Control environment to reduce misperceptions and sensory stimuli.
- Instruct care givers in techniques to avoid violent responses from client (e.g., explaining activities, not approaching from back of client, ceasing activity if client starts to become agitated).
- Protect client from harming self and others; observe, remove objects that could be potentially harmful, place in seclusion or restraints if ordered and necessary.
- Ensure care givers do not respond in aggressive manner or make threats; they need to understand client's inability to control behavior and importance of calm approach.
- Adhere to treatment plan to eliminate or minimize underlying cause; administer medications as ordered.

Evaluation
- Client is free from violent outbursts and behavior.
- Client experiences elimination or reduction of causative/contributing factors.
- Client learns new coping behaviors.

Possible Related Nursing Diagnoses
Altered thought processes
Anxiety
Fear
High risk for injury
Ineffective individual coping
Powerlessness
Sensory-perceptual alteration

RECOMMENDED READINGS

Atchley R: *Social forces in later life,* Belmont, CA; 1988, Wadsworth.
Bahr SJ, Peterson ET: *Aging and the family,* Lexington, MA; 1989, Lexington Books.
Baldwin B: Family caregiving: trends and forecasts, *Geriatr Nurs* 11:172, 1990.
Baumogen VE, Hien KF: *Helping the aging family: a guide for professionals,* Glenview, IL, 1990, Scott, Foresman.

Clark CC: *The nurse as group leader,* ed 2, New York, 1987, Springer.
McGuire FA, Boyd R: Leisure in later life. In Baines EM, editor: *Perspectives on gerontological nursing,* Newbury Park, CA, 1991, SAGE.
Schultz R, Ewen RB: *Adult development and aging: myths and emerging realities,* New York, 1988, Macmillan.

11

Sexuality and Reproduction

S exuality encompasses more than physical stimulation and pleasure. Sexual identity can determine roles, expectations, and self-worth; it can bring pleasure, warmth, and meaning to an older person's life and offset the many losses that accompany aging.

Sexual function is not normally lost with age, yet attitudes and expectations imply that older adults are not interested in or capable of sex. Few advertisements or media programs portray the elderly as vivacious sexual beings. Older persons who acquire intimate friends or housemates of the opposite sex are often ridiculed or scorned. Homosexual orientation among the elderly is afforded little attention.

No significant change takes place in sexual attitudes and behaviors with age. Sexual enjoyment neither increases nor decreases. Masturbation, homosexuality, multiple partners, infidelity, and other practices throughout adulthood usually extend into old age.

Institutions deter intimacy by separating married couples, discouraging intimate relationships, and reporting residents' sexual behavior to family members. Older couples' privacy is frequently invaded without thought that intimacy may be interrupted.

Gerontologic nurses should be informed of the realities of

sexual function in late life so that they may effectively educate clients and clarify misconceptions. Sexual responses of the older woman include the following:

- Unchanged clitoral response to stimulation
- Nipple erections during sexual excitement and possibly several hours after orgasm
- Less flushing of the skin (result of a superficial vasocongestive skin response)
- Reduced response of labia minoris and majoris
- Decreased vaginal lubrication
- Decreased vaginal wall expansion
- Similar orgasm and vaginal contractions, although vaginal contractions are shorter
- Urinary frequency and urgency after intercourse
- Nipple erection possible for hours after intercourse

Sexual responses of the older man include the following:

- Erection takes longer to achieve, requires more direct physical stimulation, and is more readily lost after interruption
- Often able to prolong time before ejaculation
- Less flushing of skin
- Orgasm similar to youthful response
- Ejaculation may be less forceful and may not occur at all during intercourse (particularly if intercourse is frequent)

❖ Generic Care Plan:
SEXUAL DYSFUNCTION

GENERAL INFORMATION

Sexual dysfunction is an impairment in the ability to experience sexual pleasure.

CAUSATIVE/CONTRIBUTING FACTORS

Male
Prostatitis: causes discomfort, interferes with ejaculation
Open type of prostatectomy: impotency

Peyronie's disease: fibrous scarring from chronic inflammation causes painful bending of penis on erection

Spinal trauma resulting in impotency

Medication, particularly antihypertensives and psychotropics

Parkinsonism: impotency

Female

Decreased estrogen level: vaginal dryness

Infection of reproductive system

Extended abstinence

Gynecologic problems: uterine prolapse, rectocele, cystocele

Both sexes

Social opposition to and/or ridicule of sexual behavior in the elderly

Illness of self or partner
> Diabetes mellitus
> Arteriosclerosis
> Parkinson's disease
> High blood pressure
> Cardiac illness
> Arthritis
> Neurologic disease

Altered body function or appearance of self or partner

Boredom, fatigue

Psychologic problems
> Depression
> Stress
> Anxiety

Lack of privacy

Unavailability of partner, prolonged sexual inactivity

Negative personal attitude toward sex (may never have found sex pleasurable or had some bad experience)

Lack of knowledge

High intake of alcohol, overeating

Joint inflexibility or pain

CLINICAL MANIFESTATIONS

Male: impotence

Female: dyspareunia (painful intercourse)

Verbalization of problems with sexuality

Frequent seeking of confirmation of desirability

NURSING PROCESS

Assessment Considerations

- Review sexual function as part of the overall evaluation of all elderly clients
- Review lifelong sexual activity (helps place client's current condition into perspective)
- Inquire about medications used and be alert to those that could affect sexual function (e.g., antihypertensives)
- Impact of illness or surgery on sexuality; changes in roles, lowered self-esteem
- Knowledge level, misinformation
- Physical evaluation
- *Females*
  - Menstrual and pregnancy history
  - Sexual interest and activity
  - Pattern of gynecologic care (professional visits and self-examination), genitalia, breasts
- *Males*
  - Sexual interest and activity
  - Self-examination of genitalia
  - Prostate status

Goal

- Client achieves desired satisfaction in the expression of own sexuality.

Nursing Interventions

- Set an accepting, nonjudgmental, and open tone when discussing sexual problems with older persons.
- Encourage open expression and discussion of sexual concerns.
- Assist in resolving sexual problems by the following actions:
  - Counseling and education as necessary
  - Arranging for comprehensive examination if an organic problem is suspected
  - Discussing realistic limitations in the face of illness
  - Seeking resources from organizations to help client compensate for disease-related sexual limitations (e.g., the Arthritis Foundation has literature demonstrating alternate sexual positions for people with severe symptoms)
  - Referring to sex counselors and clinics if specific therapy is indicated

- Educate client about real sexual changes accompanying age; clarify myths that may exist.
- Stress physical care in maintenance of sexual function:
   Genital hygiene
   Regular medical examination (gynecologic and prostate)
   Self-examination (breasts, penis, scrotum)
   Prevention and recognition of infections
   Complications of chronic diseases
- Reinforce client's sexual identity by acknowledging and assisting with efforts to look attractive.
- Respect the privacy of clients; provide appropriate place and uninterrupted time to be alone with partner.
- Treat intimate relationships among older persons with dignity and seriousness.
- Be alert to clients' and significant others' comments and behavior that may indicate a concern regarding sexual functioning or satisfaction.

Evaluation
- Client expresses satisfaction with own sexuality.
- Client learns methods to obtain sexual gratification.

Possible Related Nursing Diagnoses
Altered family processes
Anxiety
Disturbance in body image or self-concept
Impaired social interaction

 Selected Health Problems Associated with SEXUAL DYSFUNCTION
Breast Cancer

GENERAL INFORMATION

Breast cancer is a malignant growth within breast tissue and a leading cause of cancer deaths in the elderly. Decreased fat and atrophy of the breasts with age may enable masses to be more easily palpated in older women. Although a problem primarily affecting women, a small percentage of all breast cancers occurs in men.

CAUSATIVE/CONTRIBUTING FACTORS

Cause unknown
Predisposing factors: family history of breast cancer, nulliparity, late menopause

CLINICAL MANIFESTATIONS

Nontender lump
Recently developed asymmetry of breasts
Dimpling, "orange-peel" skin
Nipple discharge, bleeding, retraction
Palpable nodular masses
Signs of advanced disease
>   Pain
>   Weight loss
>   Weakness

ADDITIONAL NURSING INTERVENTIONS
TO INCORPORATE INTO GENERIC CARE PLAN

- Instruct all female clients in monthly breast self-examination; link examination date to regular monthly event to aid client in remembering to perform examination (e.g., when Social Security check is received or utility bill paid).
- Recommend annual mammography.
- Obtain prompt medical evaluation when suspicious mass or breast change is discovered.
- Ensure client understands treatment alternatives if malignancy is present.
- If surgery is performed:
>   Observe for complication of lymphedema of arm (e.g., swelling of arm on operative side).
>   Initiate rehabilitative measures such as exercises to promote full range of motion to arm and shoulders.
>   Arrange for prosthesis as soon as possible.
- Offer emotional support to client and partner:
>   Encourage ventilation of feelings.
>   Clarify misconceptions.
>   Link with cancer support group (e.g., Reach to Recovery).
- Reinforce importance of regular follow-up.

Senile vaginitis

GENERAL INFORMATION

Older women are at risk for vaginitis because of age-related changes that predispose to infection, such as gradual atrophy of vaginal tissues, decrease in vaginal lubrication, and reduced size of uterus and cervix.

CAUSATIVE/CONTRIBUTING FACTORS

Age-related changes
Trauma
Poor hygiene

CLINICAL MANIFESTATIONS

Vaginal itching
Soreness, burning, redness of vaginal canal
Vaginal discharge

ADDITIONAL NURSING INTERVENTIONS
TO INCORPORATE INTO GENERIC CARE PLAN

- Question and educate clients at risk (many older women view vaginitis as a younger women's problem and may not associate their symptoms with this condition).
- Instruct client in proper hygiene.
- Reinforce treatment plan.
- Do not assume client understands that topical medications should not be ingested; give specific instructions.
- If douche is prescribed, emphasize importance of measuring water temperature to prevent burning to fragile vaginal tissue.

Impotency

GENERAL INFORMATION

Impotency is an inability to obtain penile erection. It can be temporary or permanent, and it can result from either organic or psychologic causes. Impotency is not normal for older men.

CAUSATIVE/CONTRIBUTING FACTORS

Depression, anxiety
Drugs (particularly antihypertensives)
Obesity
Alcoholism
Diabetes
Neurologic disorders

CLINICAL MANIFESTATION

Partial or complete inability of penis to become erect

ADDITIONAL NURSING INTERVENTIONS
TO INCORPORATE INTO GENERIC CARE PLAN

- Assist with identification and treatment of underlying cause.
- Ensure client understands realities of condition; counsel as to whether or not return of potency can be anticipated.
- Assist client and partner in achieving sexually satisfying relationship:

    Emphasize importance of patience and continuing efforts.
    Discuss forms of sexual gratification other than intercourse (e.g., touching, masturbation, oral sex).
    Discuss the role of performance anxiety and how it affects one's physiologic responses.

- Refer client for penile implant, sex therapy, or other treatment as appropriate.

RECOMMENDED READINGS

Eliopoulos C: Assessment of sexual function. In Eliopoulos C, editor: *Health assessment of the older adult,* ed 2, Redwood City, CA, 1990: Addison-Wesley.

Steinke EE: Sexuality in aging. In Baines EM, editor: *Perspectives on gerontological nursing,* Newbury Park, CA, 1991, SAGE.

Walz T, Blum N: *Sexual health in later life,* Lexington, MA, 1987, DC Health.

Wisby M, Denny MS, Kissane K: For men only, *Geriatr Nurs* 12(1):26, 1991.

12

❖ Values and Beliefs

M ost individuals possess a set of beliefs that guide their lives. These beliefs give a reason for existence, hope, and a sense of right and wrong. One's attitudes toward growing old and managing health and illness can be influenced by the beliefs held. For example, a different level of acceptance accompanies a belief that the ills of the aged are God's will and must be accepted than would exist if one believed individuals control their own destinies and must use every resource available to fight illness.

Values and beliefs do not dissolve when a person becomes aged or ill. In fact, they may become more important than ever. Nurses must be familiar with various religious beliefs and philosophies so that they respect, advocate, and support practices consistent with them.

FACING DEATH

As aging people witness increasing numbers of contemporaries dying and experience more health problems themselves they become acutely aware of their own mortality. Such awareness that death is a reality and may soon be approaching often stimulates older persons to evaluate the meaning of their lives. They may be interested in putting their lives in order, resolving conflicts with family and friends, planning for the distribution of estates, and ensuring the well-being of loved ones. Individuals' lifelong patterns of dealing with problems will influence how they face the recognition that their years of life are shrinking. The pragmatic father who began his child's college fund before that child was born may have developed a detailed will describing the disposition of all his assets and written an advance directive, whereas the person who lived one day at a time and retreated from problems may not give any considerations to his or her own mortality. There is no single style of facing death. People will die as they have lived.

A terminal illness makes death an inescapable reality. This profound experience may trigger a variety of emotional reactions. Dr. Elizabeth Kübler-Ross (1969) gave insight into the reactions

---

BOX 12-1   Emotional Reactions to Dying

DENIAL
By avoiding the topic of death the client can gain time to mobilize defenses. It is important to allow the client this time and not force discussions regarding the terminal nature of the illness or death.

ANGER
Hostility and rage are felt as the client begins to think about the reality of death and experience bitterness that it is happening. Frequently, family and staff closest to the client receive this displaced anger. The client needs to release tension by venting this feeling and the most helpful approach for nurses is to accept this anger without judgment or being personally hurt.

BARGAINING
The client may try to extend life by seeking compromises or trade-offs. Many times, bargaining is done through prayers. Support is needed during this period, as well as protection that the client doesn't get taken advantage of by quacks and others who offer unrealistic cures or life extensions.

DEPRESSION
A form of mourning occurs as the patient considers the losses that will be faced. The client will need support and the presence of others—even if this means sitting in silence for extended periods of time. Human contact through hand holding and massages can be especially helpful.

ACCEPTANCE
As the client comes to terms with death he or she may be able to discuss it and begin to address issues openly. Support is needed as the client openly expresses feelings and discusses plans.

of dying individuals when she categorized the stages of death: denial, anger, bargaining, depression, and acceptance (Box 12-1). Not all dying persons experience every stage, nor will they progress through the stages in an orderly manner. Family members and care givers also may experience similar reactions as they cope with the loss of the dying person.

The realization that death is imminent can be devastating and emotionally crippling if one feels life has been useless or insignificant. By helping the elderly to evaluate their lives (Figure 12-1) nurses can help older adults to work through unresolved

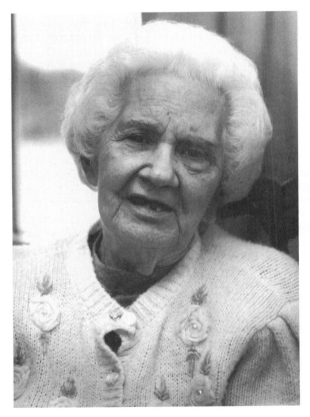

FIGURE 12-1 Acceptance of choices and life as lived is the key to inner peace in late life.

feelings and recognize accomplishments. The result can be enhanced self-esteem, satisfaction with one's life, and a clearer understanding of the "unfinished business" that needs to be resolved in one's remaining life.

The process of *life review* has been described as an essential part of letting go and preparing for death. Nurses can support efforts at life review by promoting reminiscence by older adults, either individually or through group activity (see Box 9-1).

Reminiscence may not be a comfortable experience for clients or nurses. It can be difficult to rekindle old anger, frustrations, guilt, disappointments, and other feelings; a variety of reactions can result. Nurses must understand that these uncomfortable reactions may need to be experienced to resolve past conflicts. Clients need support during this experience and reassurance that they managed situations in the best manner that they could at the time. Strengths and accomplishments should be reinforced, and shortcomings need to be forgiven. The more the individual can accept the totality of his or her life, the successes and failures, the more integration occurs and the less despair one feels. Acceptance of choices and life as lived is the key to inner peace.

❖ Generic Care Plan:
SPIRITUAL DISTRESS

GENERAL INFORMATION

Spiritual distress is a state in which beliefs or value systems are disturbed or at risk of being disturbed. Illness, multiple losses, and facing death require the individual to rely on his or her spiritual beliefs and practices to maintain the strength and courage to continue living. When people begin to question "Why me?" and "What's the meaning of this event?" they are experiencing a conflict between their beliefs and the reality of the situation. Spiritual distress results. The individual's beliefs and values no longer provide a framework for understanding life and one's purpose and place on earth. Nurses need to promote spiritual integrity to strengthen the client's ability to manage life's challenges and problems.

CAUSATIVE/CONTRIBUTING FACTORS

Physical illness
  Altered body image
  Loss of function
  Pain
Terminal illness
Change in meaningful relationships
  Illness or loss of significant other
  Own limitation in continuing relationship
Limitations imposed by situation or others
  Hospitalization, institutionalization
  Isolation, confinement
  Opposition or interference by care givers, family
Conflicts between religious practices and prescribed treatment
  Special diet
  Medications, transfusions, intravenous lines
  Life-sustaining measures

CLINICAL MANIFESTATIONS

Anger, resentment over suffering or quality of life
Anxiety, fear
Guilt
Inability to practice usual religious rituals
Discouragement
Verbalization of doubts or concerns about beliefs
Request for visits from clergy
Questioning credibility of belief system (e.g., "Why is God letting this happen to me?")

NURSING PROCESS

Assessment Considerations

- Religious beliefs, practices, preferences; determine the following:
  Type of belief, for example, God, Buddha, man is in control of own destiny (Box 12-2)
  Desire to have specific member of clergy or religious organization contacted

Text continued on p. 329.

BOX 12-2   Major Religions: Implications for Nursing

CHRISTIANITY

Christianity, the largest religion in the world, is based on the teachings of Jesus. It is believed that God manifested himself through his Son Jesus, who lived on earth and died on the cross as an atonement for the sins of humanity. Christmas is celebrated as the birth and Easter as the resurrection of Jesus. The Bible is the chief literature of Christianity. Christianity is divided into various groups with different practices: the traditional religions of the Roman Catholic and Eastern Orthodox churches and the reform religions of Prostestantism and various independent churches.

Catholic — Believe in the Pope as the head of the church on earth. Express their faith mainly in formulated creeds, such as the Apostles' Creed. Observe the sacraments of Mass, baptism of infants, confirmation, penance, matrimony, holy orders, and extreme unction (anointing individuals just before death). Attend Mass on Sundays and holy days and confess their sins to a priest at least once yearly. Fast from meat on Ash Wednesday and Good Friday; fasting during Lent and on Fridays is optional, although it is observed by some. Accept modern medical treatment. May want to have visit by priest when ill for confession and communion.

Eastern Orthodox — Includes *Greek, Serbian, Russian,* and *other orthodox churches.* Believe in Divine Liturgy, symbolism of bread and wine for body and blood of Christ. Recognize Jesus as head of church. Reject authority of the Pope; believe Holy Spirit proceeds from Father (rather than Father and Son). Priests do not need to practice celibacy. Church services are usually longer than other religions and performed in language of local people. Use icons (sacred pictures) to decorate church; sacraments are performed behind a screened area. Follow different calendar for religious feasts (e.g., Easter may fall on different date than that observed by other Christian groups). Fast during Lent and before Communion. Accept modern medical treatment. Holy unction administered to sick but not always as last rites. Pray for the dead and believe that the dead look after those on earth.

Protestant — Divided into several different churches that have various practices. Began as revolt within Catholic Church; reject authority of the Pope. *Lutherans, Methodists, and Presbyterians* support modern medical treatment, practice communion and last rites. Pres-

BOX 12-2   Major Religions: Implications for Nursing— cont'd

Protestant— cont'd

byterians believe worship of God should be done in simple, dignified way.

Baptists and *Pentecostals* view illness as a form of punishment or an act by Satan. They are baptized as adults. Against consumption of alcohol, coffee, tea, pork, or tobacco. Some may display some resistance to modern medical treatment and instead prefer divine healing through laying on of hands.

Episcopalians may abstain from meat on Fridays and fast during Lent and before Communion. May practice spiritual healing as adjunct to modern medicine. Practice confession, Communion, and last rites.

Other Christian Religions

Christian Scientists (Church of Christ, Scientist) observe a religion based on the use of faith for healing and may oppose traditional medical treatments such as medications, intravenous lines, transfusions, and special therapies. Believe sickness and sin are not real but only *appear* to humans; therefore it is possible to heal humans of sickness, sin, and limitations. Utilize Christian Science practitioners who devote their lives to healing. May be less likely to accept disease as incurable.

Friends (Quakers) believe God is personal and real, not a figment of imagination, true religion is experiential, and any believer can achieve communion with Christ without the use of trained clergy or church rituals. There is no clerical hierarchy. Do not use alcohol. May oppose the use of medications. Do not believe in an afterlife.

Jehovah's Witnesses take most ideas from the New Testament Book of Revelation. Believe Christ will return when there will be a great battle at Armageddon between him and the forces of evil; the evil will be defeated and for the next 1000 years Christ will reign on earth. Worship in Kingdom halls rather than churches. There are no special ministers; each member is considered to be a minister of the gospel and must house visit and distribute their literature every month. Believe other churches are controlled by the devil. Do not eat meats containing blood unless blood has been drained; do not consume alcohol or

Continued.

BOX 12-2   Major Religions: Implications for Nursing— Cont'd

tobacco. Oppose modern medical treatments, such as transfusions.

Mennonites believe in nonviolence, a simple and plain dress style, and a simple life-style. They are baptized as adults. They may resist medications.

Mormons (Church of Jesus Christ of Latter Day Saints) have no professional clergy; believe any male member can lead service. Do not consume coffee, tea, or alcohol or use tobacco; may restrict meat intake and fast once each month. Believe illness results from violation of God's commandments or failure to follow laws of health. May oppose modern medical treatment and use divine healing through laying on of hands.

Seventh-Day Adventists advocate principles of healthful living through diet, exercise, and philanthropic outlook. Saturday, the seventh day of the week, is their holy day. Treatment may be opposed on the Sabbath. May practice divine healing. Oppose consuming coffee, tea, or alcohol; may not eat meat and shellfish. May desire baptism or communion when seriously ill.

Unitarians represent a highly liberal branch of Christianity. Believe in God as a single being rather than belief in the doctrine of the Trinity. Accept modern medical treatment. Believe individuals are responsible for their own health status. Accept cremation.

JUDAISM

Judaism, a religion that has been practiced since the time of Moses (1500-1200 BC), recognizes one universal God (Yahweh) and believes that Jews were specially chosen to receive God's law. Jews observe their Sabbath from sundown Friday to nightfall Saturday, during which there is attendance at the synagogue and a Sabbath meal. On the Sabbath, Orthodox Jews will not work (testimony to God having created the universe in six days and having rested on the seventh) and may refuse nonemergent medical treatment. Religious services are led by a rabbi who acts more as a teacher than a traditional minister.

There are three branches of Judaism. **Orthodox** Jews believe in the divinely inspired five Books of Moses, also known as the Torah, and strictly adhere to the traditions of Judaism. Within this branch are the Hasidic Jews who subscribe to a traditional dress style. **Reform** Jews are more liberal; they call syn-

BOX 12-2   Major Religions: Implications for Nursing—Cont'd

agogues temples and may ordain female rabbis. ***Conservative*** Jews are between Orthodox and Reform Jews; they attempt to apply Jewish laws to daily life.

Essential to Jewish practice is the observance of laws and customs. These include observance of dietary restrictions that only kosher (fit) foods be eaten; pork and shellfish are forbidden, as is the mixing of dairy and meat products at the same meal. Meat must be butchered according to special rabbinical rituals. Circumcision is another practice of Jews and consists of cutting off the foreskin of the penis; this gives special identity to Jews and welcomes the infant into the religious community.

Besides the Sabbath observance, Jews observe other special celebrations. These are viewed as not merely memorials to ancient events, but as opportunities for Jewish people to relive and renew their connection with the spiritual/historical events that make up their heritage; these include the following:

Rosh Hashanah (New Year): Two-day celebration that occurs in September or October (based on the Jewish lunar calendar); a time when Jews examine their lives

Yom Kippur (Day of Atonement): considered the most holy day, in which Jews fast from food and water and repent their sins of the previous year; Orthodox Jews may not wash, engage in sex, bathe, or wear leather shoes

Sukkoth (Feast of Tabernacles): celebrated 5 days after Yom Kippur; weeklong feast commemorating God's providence during Israelites' sojourn in the desert; families often build tentlike structures decorated with harvest fruits in which they may eat and sleep

Hanukkah (Festival of Lights): celebrated in December; commemorates restoration of the Temple after it had been desecrated by the Syrians in 160 BC; during this celebration a candelabra holding eight candles is used in which an additional candle is lighted each day of the celebration

Purim: occurs in February or March; celebrates the deliverance of the Jewish people from a plot to annihilate them through the reading of the Book of Esther; Jews may fast on day preceding

Pesach (Passover): occurs in spring; celebrated through the seder, a ceremonial meal in which wines, unleavened bread (matzo), and other special foods are used symbolically during the reading of the Haggadah, the story of the Jews' escape from Egypt

Shavous: Two-day holiday, 7 weeks after Passover, that celebrates the receiving of the Torah on Mt. Sinai

Jews support modern medical treatments. On death, the body is washed and

Continued.

BOX 12-2 Major Religions: Implications for Nursing— Cont'd

burial occurs as soon as possible thereafter. During the time of death and burial, mourners show their sorrow by wearing a torn garment or a symbolic black cloth. After burial, mourners enter a 7-day period of *shiv'ah* in which they avoid work and social functions.

Jews believe that after death the person stands in judgment before God and is punished or rewarded, depending on the life he or she has lived on earth.

ISLAM (MUSLIM)
Islam is the world's third largest monotheistic (belief in one God) religion. It was founded by the prophet Mohammed who was born in Mecca about 570 AD. Mohammed was a human messenger or prophet who was used by God to communicate God's word. Muslims believe Jesus was another prophet who will return at the end of the world to guide the faithful. The Koran represents the Word of God and is the scripture followed by Islamics. There is no organized priesthood. Friday is the Sabbath.

Islam is divided into two groups: the *Sunni muslims,* who represent most Islamics, and *Shi'ite muslims.*

Islamics eat no pork and abstain from alcohol. Cleanliness is an important part of their practice. They may pray five times daily, facing toward Mecca. They accept medical treatments if these do not violate religious practices. Illness is seen as God's will.

Dying Islamics may want to confess. On death, the family prepares the body and the body must face Mecca. Organ donation, cremation, and autopsy (unless required by law) are prohibited.

BUDDHISM
Buddhism is an offshoot of Hinduism and has many followers in the East. Buddhists believe enlightenment is found through individual meditation rather than communal worship. Buddhists see the root of all suffering in life as an outgrowth of desire for false selfhood and other desires. They strive to achieve a form of liberation and enlightenment known as *nirvana.* The moral code that leads to nirvana is the *Eightfold Path:*

Right understanding: life is understood as changing and painful
Right thoughts: thoughts of goodwill and nonharming
Right speech: avoidance of lies, slander, gossip, harsh words
Right action: refraining from killing, stealing, harmful sexual behavior
Right means of livelihood: dealing morally with tasks of daily life, avoidance of jobs involving weapons, intoxicating drinks, slaughter of animals
Right effort: resisting impulses that generate greed and violence
Right mindfulness: attention to what is being done at the moment and the changing realities of life

BOX 12-2 Major Religions: Implications for Nursing—Cont'd

Right concentration: concentration on right goals and thoughts through the use of meditation

Buddhists are vegetarians and abstain from alcohol and tobacco. They may oppose medications and refuse treatments on holy days. Euthanasia is allowed in hopeless situations. Illness may be viewed as a test of strength that aids in one's development; meditation may be an important part of the healing process.

HINDUISM

Hinduism may be the world's oldest religion and is the religion of most of India's inhabitants. Hinduism has no scriptures, no fixed doctrines, and no common worship. Most Hindus believe everything is part of one reality, although some worship many Indian gods.

Two key concepts of Hindu belief are *karma* (belief that every person is born into a position in life based on deeds of previous life) and *samsara* (reincarnation). Among Hindus there can be different types of beliefs such as the protection of cows (symbolizes human obligation to protect the weak or oppressed) and nonviolence.

Health and dietary practices parallel those of Buddhists. Illness may be viewed as a result of sin from another life. Cremation is supported.

From Eliopoulos C: Understanding religious differences, *Long Term Care Educator* 4(12), 1993. © Health Education Network, 11104 Glen Arm Road, Glen Arm, MD 21057.

Type of measures to assist in supporting religious practices, for example, taking client to chapel Sunday mornings, obtaining a Bible, providing 15 minutes of privacy each morning
- Beliefs that could conflict with health practices or treatment plan, for example, refusal of medications, dietary practices

Goal
- Client maintains religious beliefs and practices to maximum degree possible.

Nursing Interventions
- Acquaint all care givers with client's needs and desires pertaining to religious beliefs; ensure care givers are nonjudgmental.
- Make necessary arrangements for continuation and support of religious practices (e.g., obtain special articles, arrange for clergy visitation, pray with client or arrange for someone else to).

- Adhere to imposed practices or restrictions unless the client has decided to violate them.
- Obtain dietary consultation or arrange for special foods to be brought from home.
- Know specific Sabbath days and respect them.
- Follow unique postmortem practices.
- Allow client to express feelings; understand that life review and a discussion of the reasons for current problems aid in putting one's life in perspective and understanding its purpose.

Evaluation
- Client expresses satisfaction with ability to maintain and practice religious beliefs.

Possible Related Nursing Diagnoses
Anxiety
Fear
Grieving
Hopelessness
Ineffective family or individual coping
Knowledge deficit
Powerlessness
Sleep pattern disturbance

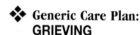

❖ Generic Care Plan: GRIEVING

GENERAL INFORMATION

Grief is the emotional reaction that follows the loss of a function or love object. Older adults experience many losses that could precipitate grieving, such as the death of a loved one or pet, the need to move from a lifelong family home, a decline in health status, and the forfeiture of important roles. The duration of the reaction varies but may last for over a year. Grief disrupts daily life and often affects physical functioning as well.

CAUSATIVE/CONTRIBUTING FACTORS

Loss of health, energy, activity
Loss of role related to family, work

Loss of financial income, altered economic status
Loss of youth, beauty
Loss of friends, family, pet (Figure 12-2)
Loss of home, alterations in living accommodations
Loss of mobility, senses
Diagnosis of terminal illness

CLINICAL MANIFESTATIONS

Somatic symptoms
    Fatigue, insomnia
    Empty feelings, lump in throat
    Hyperventilation
    Anorexia
Psychologic symptoms
    Shock, disbelief, denial, avoidance
    Anger, mental discomfort, irritability
    Bargaining, loss of faith, "why me?"
    Sorrow, crying, depression
Behavioral symptoms
    Complaining, demanding
    Hostility, rage, bitterness
    Displaced anger onto staff, family
    Avoidance of feelings by using distractions (e.g., television, busywork)
    Discouragement, giving up

NURSING PROCESS

Assessment Considerations
- Exact nature of the loss(es) and when occurred
- Meaning of the loss to the individual
- Realistic perception of loss or potential loss
- Social and cultural perceptions of the meaning of death, life after death, and how to prepare for death
- Spritual beliefs and practices; desire for religious counsel
- Stage of grief
- Physical reactions, need for assistance in activities of daily living
- Available support system

Goal
- Client copes with the loss or impending death by adaptively completing each stage of the grief and mourning process.

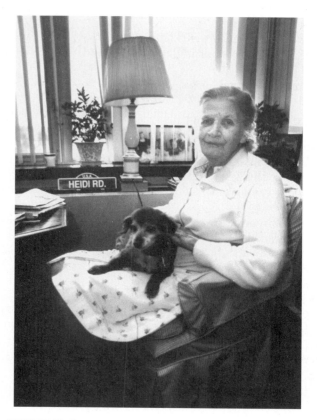

FIGURE 12-2 Significant grieving can result from the loss of one's pet.

Nursing Interventions

- Encourage open expression of feelings but do not force discussion beyond what the client is ready and willing to face.
- Encourage hope, assist client in making plans, but do not foster unrealistic goals and beliefs.
- Answer questions honestly, provide information about present status as needed.
- Be aware that the client may insist on second and third opinions about prognosis or claim there is a mix-up; this is part of the denial phase.
- Allow denial as long as necessary since it allows the client time to mobilize personal defenses.

- Be sensitive to changing emotional states; client may fluctuate between stages.
- Recognize the stages of anger and bargaining and how they are manifested: displaced feelings, "why me?", trying to secure more time to finish business.
- Do not take client's anger toward staff personally; displacement of anger and frustrations is common.
- Provide comfort, physical contact, and frequent interactions.
- Pay particular attention to physical needs; feed if necessary, provide protection and comfort, introduce preventive measures to maintain nutrition and elimination patterns.
- Give medication as needed for pain, anxiety, depression.
- Be alert to new physical and emotional symptoms and evaluate their relationship to stage of grief.
- Be sensitive to the emotional needs of family and friends; suggest counseling if appropriate.
- Prepare client and family for the inevitable depression that follows recognition that all attempts at bargaining are futile and one has to accept the loss of relationships, unfulfilled dreams, and life itself.
- Schedule time with client to discuss how he or she is preparing for death and saying good-bye to people, things, and life.
- Encourage client to resolve unfinished business and conflicts with loved ones, plan disposition of estate, and make a will.
- Recognize the problem of loneliness for elderly people and their ambivalent desire to end the pain and isolation vs. the instinctive desire to live and the fear of death.
- Assist the family in funeral preparations by referring to appropriate resources for arrangements, insurance, Social Security benefits, and so on.
- Assist family in ventilating feelings and continue to support family after client's death.
- Refer survivors to support groups and counseling as appropriate.
- Suggest professional help for anyone suffering from dysfunctional grief.

Evaluation
- Client speaks realistically about loss with an acceptance of consequences.
- Client exhibits minimal denial, anger, and sorrow.

Possible Related Nursing Diagnoses
Altered family processes
Anxiety
Hopelessness
Ineffective individual coping
Sleep pattern disturbance
Spiritual distress

RECOMMENDED READINGS

Benoliel JQ: Multiple meanings of death for older adults. In Baines EM, editor: *Perspectives on gerontological nursing*, Newbury Park, CA, 1991, SAGE.

Gass KA, Chang AS: Appraisals of bereavement, coping, resources, and psychosocial health dysfunction in widows and widowers, *Nurs Res* 38:31, 1989.

Herth K: Relationship of hope, coping styles, concurrent losses, and setting to grief resolution in the elderly widow(er), *Res Nurs Health* 13:109, 1990.

Koenig HG, Smiley M, Gonzales JAP: *Religion, health and aging*, New York, 1988, Greenwood.

Kübler-Ross E: *On death and dying*, New York, 1969, Macmillan.

Reker GT: Meaning and purpose in life and well-being: a life-span perspective, *J Gerontol Nurs* 42(1):44, 1987.

Rhymes JA: Clinical management of the terminally ill, *Geriatrics* 46(2): 57, 1991.

Ross HK: Lesson of life, *Geriatr Nurs* 11(6):274, 1990.

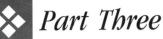

Part Three

Special
Issues
in
Gerontologic
Nursing
Care

13

❖ Drugs: Special Considerations in the Elderly

A n inescapable responsibility of gerontologic nursing is to ensure that older adults have more benefits than adverse effects from the medications they use. This is a significant concern because of the following:

- *Older adults consume a large volume of drugs.* Although they represent 12% of the total population, the elderly receive nearly one third of all drugs prescribed in the United States. A majority of older persons use at least one drug daily, with the more typical situation being several drugs each day.
- *Drugs behave differently in older adults.* Advanced age causes differences in pharmacokinetics (the absorption, distribution, metabolism, and excretion of drugs) and pharmacodynamics (the biologic and therapeutic effects of drugs at the site of action or target organ) (Table 13-1).
- *Older adults use drugs with serious side effects.* In order of use, the most common drugs consumed by the elderly are as follows:

  Cardiovascular agents
  Antihypertensives

TABLE 13-1 Age-Related Changes Affecting Drug Therapy in the Elderly

Change	Impact	Nursing measures
Drier mucous membrane of oral cavity	Tablets and capsules may stick to roof or sides of mouth and not be swallowed; can dissolve in and irritate mouth	Offer fluids before drug administration to moisten mouth and ample fluids during administration. Inspect mouth or advise client to inspect mouth for any tablet or capsule that may not have been swallowed (dentures and reduced sensations may cause client to be unaware of presence of medication). Unless contraindicated, break large tablets to facilitate swallowing.
Decreased circulation to lower bowel and vagina; lower body temperature	Suppositories require longer time to melt and risk being expelled undissolved	Explore possibility of using alternative route. Allow longer time for suppository to melt. Check/advise client to check suppository has melted before getting out of bed to resume activities.
Decreased tissue elasticity; reduced muscle mass and activity	Poor seal of tissues after injection, oozing; poor absorption	Use upper, outer quadrant of buttocks for intramuscular injections and rotate sites. Use Z-track injection technique for injections to facilitate sealing. Cleanse any medication that has oozed on skin.
Decreased pain sensation	Infection or other problem at injection site may not be detected	Check injection sites regularly.
Decreased cardiac efficiency	Greater risk of circulatory overload during intravenous administration of medications	Monitor intravenous drip closely. Observe for signs of circulatory overload (e.g., rise in blood pressure, rapid respirations, coughing, shortness of breath).

Less gastric acid	Slower absorption of drugs that require low gastric pH	Ensure gastric acid is not further reduced by other drugs (e.g., antacids).
Increase in adipose tissue compared to lean body mass; decreased cardiac output	Drugs stored in adipose tissue (lipid-soluble drugs) have increased tissue concentrations and decreased plasma concentrations and accumulate and remain in body for longer duration; plasma levels of drugs can increase while less is deposited in reservoirs (particularly true of water-soluble drugs)	Ensure dosages are age adjusted. Become familiar with adverse effects of drugs administered and observe for these effects.
Reduced serum albumin levels	Administering several protein-bound drugs together can cause drugs to compete for same protein molecules; some drugs may not effectively bind and be less effective	Advise physician of other protein-bound drugs client is taking when new protein-bound drug is prescribed; highly protein-bound drugs include acetazolamide, amitriptyline, cefazolin, chlordiazepoxide, chlorpromazine, cloxacillin, digitoxin, furosemide, hydralazine, nortriptyline, phenylbutazone, phenytoin, propranolol, rifampin, salicylates, spironolactone, sulfisoxazole, and warfarin. Ensure serum albumin level is evaluated along with blood level of drug (if serum albumin level is low, client has greater risk for becoming toxic despite normal or low blood levels of drug).
Reduced number of functioning nephrons; decreased glomerular filtration rate; reduced blood flow	Biologic half-life extended; drugs take longer to be filtered from body; increased risk of adverse reactions	Ensure age-adjusted dosages are prescribed for drugs excreted through renal system.

Analgesics
Antiarthritic agents
Sedatives
Tranquilizers
Laxatives
Antacids

These drugs carry risks that can threaten the health and well being of older persons, such as altered mental status, lightheadedness, dizziness, and fluid and electrolyte imbalances.

To effectively safeguard older clients, nurses must become familiar with the unique ways drugs behave in the elderly (see Table 13-1), the side effects associated with commonly used drugs (Table 13-2), and nursing interventions that maximize the benefits and minimize the risks associated with drug therapy.

ASSESSMENT CONSIDERATIONS

- Determine if nonpharmacologic approaches can solve or control the problem for which the drug is being used, for example:

    Warm milk and a back rub instead of a sedative

    Coffee or cranberry juice instead of a diuretic

    Warm soaks or position changes instead of an analgesic

    Dietary change instead of an antacid or laxative

    Diversional activity instead of an antipsychotic

- Ensure the lowest possible dosage is prescribed:

    The longer biologic half-life of most drugs in older persons warrants lower dosages.

    Dosage must be individualized based on body size and known organ function.

- Review other drugs being used for potential interactions.

- Keep a drug reference handy; with the growing number and changing knowledge of drugs it is unrealistic to expect to commit all drug facts to memory.

- Obtain specific guidelines for use of PRN medications and use them appropriately.

- Request that orders state the conditions for use (e.g., for shoulder pain, for temperature above 100°F).

- If client self-administers drugs, evaluate his or her capacity to do so (e.g., motor dexterity to manipulate container, knowledge, memory, judgment, vision, tendency to abuse drug).

TABLE 13-2   Side Effects of Selected Drugs

	Abnormal bruising and bleeding	Acid-base imbalance	Acute excitement	Agitation	Anaphylactic reaction	Anemias	Anorexia	Anxiety	Bone marrow depression	Breast enlargement with milk formation	Confusion	Convulsions	Delirium	Depression	Diarrhea	Disorientation	Dizziness	Drug fever	Dysrhythmias	Edema	Eye rolling	Fainting	Fluctuating blood glucose levels
Acetaminophen	x				x	x																	
Amitriptyline				x					x	x	x						x	x	x			x	x
Antacids		x																		x			
Chloral hydrate													x										
Chlordiazepoxide			x								x			x			x					x	
Chlorpromazine									x	x	x									x			
Diazepam			x								x						x						
Digoxin											x					x							
Fluphenazine				x					x								x						
Haloperidol				x	x	x	x		x	x					x	x	x		x				x
Hydrochlorothiazide				x		x			x								x	x					
Insulin											x												x
Isoniazid									x	x				x									x
Methyldopa					x																		
Perphenazine									x					x									
Phenobarbital							x		x		x					x	x	x					
Phenytoin							x		x		x						x	x					
Potassium chloride																x							
Reserpine	x								x	x													
Rifampin							x									x	x						
Theophylline								x			x					x	x		x				
Thioridazine			x				x		x	x	x	x											
Trifluoperazine			x								x						x						
Trihexyphenidyl											x						x						

Continued.

TABLE 13-2   Side Effects of Selected Drugs—Cont'd

	Gastrointestinal disturbances	Hair loss	Hallucinations	Hangover effect	Headache	Hepatitis	Hives	Hypertension	Hypotension	Impaired renal function	Increased appetite	Indigestion	Inflamed pancreas	Intestinal obstruction	Irritation of tongue	Jaundice	Kidney stone formation	Lethargy	Lowered resistance to infection	Low-grade fever	Muscle spasms
Acetaminophen							x														
Amitriptyline			x		x	x						x			x						
Antacids								x		x				x		x					
Chloral hydrate				x		x						x									
Chlordiazepoxide			x														x		x		
Chlorpromazine						x			x		x									x	x
Diazepam			x																		
Digoxin					x			x									x				
Fluphenazine					x	x															x
Haloperidol		x			x											x					
Hydrochlorothiazide	x				x	x							x								
Insulin																					
Isoniazid	x				x																
Methyldopa								x										x			
Perphenazine					x	x	x														x
Phenobarbital				x		x	x														
Phenytoin					x	x			x												x
Potassium chloride	x																				
Reserpine																					
Rifampin	x				x		x														
Theophylline					x																
Thioridazine			x			x															
Trifluoperazine																				x	x
Trihexyphenidyl																					

Nausea	Nightmares	Palpitations	Parkinson-like disorders	Peripheral neuritis	Rash	Reduced platelets	Reduced white blood cell count	Restlessness	Sexual impairment	Sleepwalking	Slurred speech	Stomach ulcers	Swelling: face and tongue	Swelling: glands	Swelling and tenderness of gums	Swelling: testicles	Swelling: vocal cords	Tachycardia	Temperature decrease	Temperature increase	Thought disturbances	Tingling sensations	Tremors	Unsteady gait	Vivid dreaming	Vision disturbances	Vomiting	Weakness
					X												X						X					
X		X	X	X	X			X					X			X								X	X		X	X
X	X																										X	
X					X						X																X	
X			X		X								X													X	X	
			X		X														X									
					X	X							X													X		
					X																					X		
					X															X								
X		X	X		X													X								X		X
					X																					X		
					X									X							X	X				X		
																												X
			X		X														X									
X					X	X						X														X		
X					X						X		X	X												X		
X					X																					X		
X			X		X				X																	X		
					X	X													X			X				X		
X					X						X							X								X		
X			X		X								X						X							X		
			X		X			X																			X	
X					X																					X		

INTERVENTIONS

- Determine the best time of day to administer the medication (e.g., diuretics in the early morning, drugs that cause drowsiness at bedtime).
- Identify special precautions for administration (e.g., relationship to meals or other drugs, the need to have an antagonist readily available).
- Give medication as prescribed, following any special instructions or precautions.

SAMPLE DRUG RECORD FOR CLIENT

Medication	Dosage	Time(s) Taken	Purpose	Special Precautions	Signs to Report

FIGURE 13-1 Sample drug record for client.

- Educate client and client's care givers about drugs and their purposes, administration, special precautions, and adverse reactions. To ensure that information will not be forgotten, write important facts on a record for the client to keep (Figure 13-1).
- Ensure that blood levels of drugs are monitored; however, be aware that toxicity can occur even with blood levels within a normal range.
- Discuss with the physician the possibility of drug holidays (Box 13-1) for the many benefits this plan provides; recognize that some physicians could have overlooked this option and may need to be reminded of the length of time the client has been using the drug.
- Evaluate if the drug is achieving the desired effect and whether side effects are occurring; document the client's response to drug therapy.
- Regularly question if the drug needs to be continued; if it is no

---

BOX 13-1   Drug Holiday

DEFINITION
The planned omission of a specific medication on one or more days each week

BENEFITS
Reduced risk of drug accumulating to toxic level in bloodstream
Increased mental alertness
Cost savings
Decreased demand on care givers' or staff's time

REQUIREMENTS
Interdisciplinary support, planning, and thorough assessment of appropriateness of client for drug holiday
Careful selection of drugs
Stabilized blood level for certain drugs
Education of client and family or care givers

DRUGS NOT USUALLY OMITTED
Antibiotics
Anticoagulants
Anticonvulsants
Antidiabetics
Ophthalmic drops

TABLE 13-3   Drug Groups Discussed in This Book

Drug group	Page location
Analgesics	269
Antacids	96
Antianginals	168
Antidysrhythmics	161
Antibiotics	70
Anticoagulants	170
Antidepressants	282
Antidiabetics	93
Antihypertensives	177
Antiinflammatories	211
Antipsychotics	241
Anxiolytics (antianxiety agents)	288
Cardiac glycosides	163
Diuretics	159
Laxatives	123

longer needed or is ineffective, relay these observations to the physician. Often, it is the nurse who sees the client on a regular basis and is best able to provide feedback concerning the client's responses to medication.

• Include the client and care givers in the evaluation process, since they are often in the best position to observe the effects of the drug.

• Educate client and care givers that nonpharmacologic measures should be used before resorting to drugs. Also, advise them to consult a pharmacist or other health care professional regarding precautions or the potential for interactions before independently using an over-the-counter drug.

NOTE: Various drug groups are discussed throughout the book with the medical problems for which they are used. Table 13-3 references the locations of these discussions.

RECOMMENDED READINGS

Bressler R, Katz MD: *Geriatric pharmacology,* New York, 1993, McGraw-Hill.

Lipton HL, Lee PL: *Drugs and the elderly: clinical, social and policy perspectives,* Stanford, CA, 1988, Stanford University.

Lowenthal DT: Clinical pharmacology. In Abrams WB, Berkow R, editors: *The Merck manual of geriatrics,* Rahway, NJ, 1990, Merck Sharp and Dohme Research Laboratories.

Miller C: When medication harms as well as helps, *Geriatr Nurs* 11(6): 301, 1990.

14

Legal and Ethical Issues in Gerontologic Nursing

etermining competence, promoting independent decision making, weighing life-sustaining treatments against a death with dignity, rationing scarce resources . . . these are some of the care-giving issues that can create special legal risks and ethical dilemmas for the elderly and their care givers. Gerontologic nurses have a professional responsibility to ensure that older clients' rights are protected. This responsibility entails more than ensuring actions fall within the legal parameters of doing things right; it also includes sensitivity to the ethical dimensions of care giving to ensure that the right things are done.

LEGAL ISSUES

As a group, the elderly are more likely than other groups to have their legal rights violated. This group is highly vulnerable for many reasons:

- The aged commonly possess health problems that make them dependent and at times less able to protect themselves.
- The aged have a higher rate of impaired cognition that could interfere with sound judgment.
- The aged tend to have fewer economic resources.
- The aged are more likely to live alone (as is the case with older women).

- The aged often are viewed as easy targets by unscrupulous individuals.

The other side of the coin is that caring for the elderly may create special legal risks for health care professionals. Altered symptomatology can delay the detection of health problems. Complications develop more easily. Responses to therapy can differ. Families may be unwilling to accept the impending death of their aged loved one and have unrealistic expectations. Reactions associated with the family's guilt, anger, and frustration concerning the care of the elder can be displaced on nursing staff. Long-term care facilities and other settings that care primarily for an aged population may rely on unlicensed nursing staff for care giving, thereby increasing the risks for the professional nurse in that setting.

Nurses must be aware of general public and private laws that all citizens must follow and ensure these are not violated in the practice setting. Further, nurses need to be familiar with and abide by administrative laws, such as regulations pertaining to specific care settings and practice acts addressing the scope and responsibilities of various professionals. Selected legal issues of interest to gerontologic nurses are described below.

Advance Directives

A living will or advance directive is a document that describes a competent individual's desires regarding future care measures.

Nursing implications

- Ask the client about the presence of an advance directive. If one exists, ensure that a copy is placed in the medical record and communicated to all staff.
- Since states can vary as to the conditions that must be met for an advance directive to be valid, check with your specific state agency on aging or legal counsel to be knowledgeable of requirements. Ensure the client's advance directive meets the conditions in the specific state. (Forms for preparing advance directives can be obtained from the Society for the Right to Die, 250 West 57th Street, New York, NY 10157.)
- Document any opinions and desires expressed by the client concerning life-sustaining measures and treatment preferences.
- Encourage clients who have not developed advance directives to consider doing so.

Assault and Battery

Every human being has the right to be free from being touched against his or her will. Assault is a threat to cause physical harm by touching a person against his or her will, whereby the person has reason to believe that the threat is real. Telling an individual that you are going to hit him or refuse to feed him constitutes assault. Battery is the act of touching a person against his or her will. Forcing a resisting person into a whirlpool bath or performing a sigmoidoscopy without consent is an example of battery.

Nursing implications

- Check that the client has granted consent for treatments, diagnostic tests, and other care measures that exceed basic care.
- Respect the client's right to refuse care.
- Ensure that care givers do not use threats to convince the client to receive care or change behavior.
- In the health care setting, allow only approved personnel to provide care.
- Do not touch coworkers or visitors without their approval. If an individual is displaying inappropriate behaviors and must be removed from a setting, obtain the assistance of security or police personnel rather than forcefully removing the person yourself.

Competency

Competency refers to the capacity of an individual to make decisions, such as granting consent or refusing care.

Nursing implications

- Clients have the right to make their own decisions regarding care unless they have been judged incompetent. Periodic confusional states, a low score on a mental status examination, eccentric behaviors, differing opinions of family members, frailty, or advanced age does not mean that a client is incompetent to make decisions.
- If there is question as to a client's competency, recommend to a family member or representative of the client that the court be petitioned to appoint a guardian who can legally make decisions for the client.
- Although the next of kin is commonly appointed guardian for an incompetent individual, there are exceptions. To safeguard practice, have someone in the agency review the legal docu-

ments naming the guardian and document this information in the client's record.

- Understand that different types of guardianship can be granted for incompetent individuals. *Guardian of property* is a limited guardianship in which the guardian can make decisions pertaining to financial matters and property of the client but cannot make decisions regarding medical treatment. *Guardian of person* is the form of guardianship in which the appointed guardian can grant consent or refuse treatment on behalf of the client.

Consent

Written consent demonstrates that the client authorizes the care giver to perform specific procedures. Most agencies have a standard consent form that clients sign on admission, authorizing routine and customary services. This consent does not cover all procedures, however. Special written consent should be obtained for the following:

- Surgery
- Use of anesthesia
- Moderate- to high-risk diagnostic procedures
- Use of cobalt or radiation
- Electroshock therapy
- Experimental drugs or procedures
- Anything other than ordinary, routine care

Nursing implications

Consent should be informed in that the client fully understands the procedure. To ensure consent is informed, the following guidelines should be observed:

- The verbal explanation and written description on the consent form should describe the name of the procedure, its purpose, the steps that will occur, alternatives, consequences, possible side effects, and risks.
- The description should be expressed on a level and in a language that the client can understand.
- A responsible professional should obtain the consent. The physician can delegate responsibility for obtaining consent, but he or she remains liable.
- If the client has been determined to be legally incompetent, obtain written consent from the legal guardian. Unless judged legally incompetent, the client has the right to grant or refuse consent. When there is doubt as to the

client's ability to understand, it may be a safeguard to obtain informed consent of the nearest relative in addition to the client (and to document specific reasons for taking this approach).

Do-Not-Resuscitate (DNR) Orders

A decision not to provide resuscitation is a medical decision and should be communicated through a physician's order. Further, since this order involves a decision regarding future care, the competent client should participate in this decision.

- Ensure that the decision against resuscitation is expressed in a medical order. Announcing the decision at a care-planning conference or writing DNR on the care plan does not suffice.
- Review and abide by your agency's policy regarding DNR orders. Make sure a mechanism exists for documenting and communicating this order to all care givers.

Documentation

The client's medical record is a legal document that must be accurate and reflect actual occurrences. All entries should contain date, time, signature, and title of person making the entry. The client's written permission must be obtained before the medical record can be shared with sources other than the agency staff.

Nursing implications

- Record all observations and care-giving activities as soon as possible.
- Remember that anything entered into the record can be used in a court of law; thus entries should be correct, timely, and conscientious.
- Document care after it was done; do not sign off all medications or treatments for the shift before doing them.
- Do not alter documentation by changing dates, changing occurrences, or destroying or replacing original entries. If an error is made in documenting, do not white out or obliterate it; instead, draw a single line through the entry, write "mistaken entry" (rather than "error"), and sign appropriately.
- Document only what you observe. If information is reported to you (e.g., that the client fell) document the source and nature of the report and your observation (e.g., "Client's roommate called for assistance, stating that she believes client fell in bath-

room. On entering bathroom, client was observed to be sitting on floor next to commode.")
- If fictious or erroneous documentation is discovered or suspected, report this to your immediate supervisor.
- In addition to documenting changes in status or symptoms, ensure this information is communicated to the physician or other appropriate care giver. Documentation does not relieve you of the responsibility for taking appropriate actions to seek timely help for the client.

Invasion of Privacy
Clients have the right to be free from public view and from having confidential information shared with others without their consent. Examples of invasion of the client's privacy could include:
- Using a photograph of the client without consent
- Sending a copy of the client's medical record to another agency without consent
- Discussing the client at a social gathering

Nursing implications
- Ensure that the client has given written consent to have personal or clinical records released to another agency.
- Do not and ensure that other staff members do not discuss the client in public areas.
- Do not allow unauthorized persons to observe or participate in the client's care without the client's consent.
- Obtain the client's permission before using photographs or identifying information in a journal article, conference presentation, report, audiovisual production, or advertisement.
- Take precautions to safeguard computer-stored information from unauthorized access.
- Respect the client's right to send and receive mail unopened, receive visitors, and use a telephone in private.

Malpractice
Health care professionals have the responsibility of ensuring that their practice is consistent with good standards of care. Malpractice can be charged if deviation from a standard of care results in harm to the client. Malpractice can arise from commission (performing a procedure inappropriately) or omission (failing to perform a procedure that should be performed). Usually, the following conditions must exist for a nurse to be liable for malpractice:

- Duty: a relationship must exist between the client and nurse in which the nurse is expected to provide service for the client
- Negligence: failure to take reasonable and prudent action that is consistent with an acceptable standard for that action
- Injury: harm results from the negligent action

Nursing implications
- Know and adhere to the approved policies and procedures of your employing agency and the standards expressed in regulations and practice acts governing your area of practice.
- Do only what you are equipped, skilled, and licensed to do.
- Review care plan and orders before giving care.
- Follow medical orders as written. Consult with the physician when an order is unclear or inappropriate. Refuse orders that appear incorrect.
- Maintain competency by keeping current on nursing practice.
- Use good judgment and follow acceptable standards of practice.
- Delegate carefully based on known capabilities of subordinates; follow up on delegated tasks.
- Identify clients before providing care.
- Monitor clients' status. Pay particular attention to the health status, vital signs, and safety (e.g., location, activities engaged in) of clients who are cognitively impaired or otherwise compromised in their ability to identify and report problems or protect themselves.
- Actively observe and listen for clients' complaints, changes in physical or mental status, and equipment malfunction; report these findings to the appropriate person as soon as possible.
- Respond promptly to complaints, incidents, and accidents.
- Keep clients informed and give explanations of care activities.
- Document accurately and thoroughly.
- Carry your own malpractice insurance to supplement that provided by your employer. Be sure to read the insurance policy carefully to ensure nursing actions are covered on and off the job (e.g., while you may be volunteering at a community health fair).

Restraints
Anything that restricts movement is considered a restraint (Figure 14-1); this could include the following:

- Protective vests
- Geri-chairs
- Safety bars
- Safety belts
- Psychotropic medications

Restraints should be used only for the physical safety of the client or other persons who are at risk of being harmed by the client's

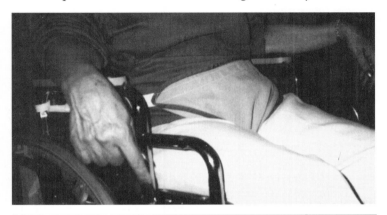

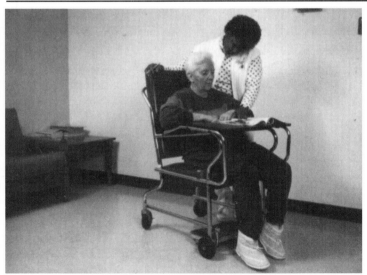

FIGURE 14-1 Pelvic restraints and geriatric chairs are forms of restraint. (From Castillo HM: *The nurse assistant in long-term care: a rehabilitative approach,* St Louis, 1992, Mosby.)

actions and not for staff convenience or to forcefully retain or discipline the client. Only after other measures have proven unsuccessful should restraints be employed. Inappropriate use of restraints can result in harm (including death) of the client and charges of battery and false imprisonment for the nurse and employing agency.

Nursing implications

- Document the specific behaviors displayed by the client that indicate the client is a risk to self or others. Describe the risk the client poses by not being restrained.
- Before using restraints attempt to manage the client with other measures. Document those measures and their effectiveness.
- Obtain a physician's order for the restraint. The order should describe the conditions for which the restraint is to be used, specific type of restraint, and duration of use.
- Closely adhere to the agency's policy and procedure for restraint use.
- Closely observe the restrained individual, and document time restraint was started, times the restraint was released or changed, response, and effectiveness.

ETHICAL ISSUES

As mentioned earlier, gerontologic nurses must be concerned with more than performing actions correctly to stay within the legal boundaries of practice; they also should ensure that ethics are incorporated into practice so that correct actions are taken with respect to what is best for the elderly.

Ethics are the beliefs people hold as to what is right and wrong, good and bad. Families and religious teachings provide individuals with basic ethics that guide their lives. In addition, ethical principles guide health care professionals, such as the following:

- *Autonomy:* nurses should work from the belief that clients have the right to make their own decisions, rather than assuming that health professionals know what is best and should decide for clients
- *Beneficence:* nurses should attempt to do good for clients
- *Nonmalfeasance:* nurses should avoid harming clients
- *Justice:* nurses should treat clients fairly
- *Veracity:* nurses should be truthful to clients

- *Fidelity:* nurses should keep commitments and honor their word to clients
- *Confidence:* nurses should respect clients' right to privacy and protect information given confidentially

These ethical principles seem reasonable, appropriate, and fairly straightforward; however, actual practice, particularly with older clients, presents circumstances that cloud the clarity of these principles, such as the following:

- An older client may be fearful of and refuse a procedure that could be lifesaving. Coercing the client into consenting to the procedure could help in keeping the client alive, but it would violate the client's right to autonomy.
- A client may have a history of falling and may avoid fall-related injury by being confined to a Geri-chair and having other moderate means of restraints used. Harm may be avoided by restraining the client, but it would be at the expense of violating the client's right to be free from restraints.
- Treating all clients fairly could be viewed as providing the same health care coverage to all older adults via Medicare. However, if a sliding scale payment method was employed, older adults who saved and invested wisely throughout their lives would bear more of a burden than those who may have had similar income but spent their money on luxury items and recreation and have no resources in old age.
- A competent client may ask about his prognosis, which professional staff members know to be poor. The client has expressed his views of wanting to arrange to commit suicide if he has no hope of improving. Being honest with the client could result in the client's decision to end his life, but it is the client's right to be informed.

Situations such as those described above can result in ethical dilemmas in which the right action to take is unclear. Gerontologic care presents, and will continue to present, many ethical dilemmas for nurses. Although not all ethical dilemmas can be neatly resolved, there are measures nurses can follow to promote an ethical nursing practice:

- Incorporate the American Nurses' Association Code of Ethics into your nursing practice; share this code with other care givers (Box 14-1).

BOX 14-1   Code for Nurses

The nurse provides services with respect for human dignity and the uniqueness of the client, unrestricted by considerations of social or economic status, personal attributes, or the nature of health problems.

The nurse safeguards the client's right to privacy by judiciously protecting information of a confidential nature.

The nurse acts to safeguard the client and the public when health care and safety are affected by the incompetent, unethical, or illegal practice of any person.

The nurse assumes responsibility and accountability for individual nursing judgments and actions.

The nurse maintains competence in nursing.

The nurse exercises informed judgment and uses individual competence and qualifications as criteria in seeking consultation, accepting responsibilities, and delegating nursing activities to others.

The nurse participates in activities that contribute to the ongoing development of the profession's body of knowledge.

The nurse participates in the profession's efforts to implement and improve standards of nursing.

The nurse participates in the profession's efforts to establish and maintain conditions of employment conducive to high quality nursing care.

The nurse participates in the profession's effort to protect the public from misinformation and misrepresentation and to maintain the integrity of nursing.

The nurse collaborates with members of the health professions and other citizens in promoting community and national efforts to meet the health needs of the public.

From American Nurses' Association: *Code for nurses with interpretive statements,* Washington, DC, 1985, American Nurses Association.

- Review your agency's policies and procedures that address ethical issues, such as advance directives, client's refusal of needed care, and disagreement among staff with treatment goals. Recommend the development of policies and procedures as needed.
- Be aware of your own value system and refrain from imposing your values on clients.
- Advocate for the protection of clients' rights.
- Ensure decisions are not made that are age biased (e.g., withholding treatment because the client is of a specific age, obtaining consent from the child rather than the older client).

- Ensure clients are not coerced into granting consent or making decisions.
- Refer ethical issues and dilemmas to the ethics committee as needed. If your agency lacks an ethics committee, recommend that one be developed. Members of this committee could include nurses, physicians, social workers, clergy, attorneys, clients, family members, trustees, and other individuals as appropriate. The activities of an ethics committee could include the following:

    Educating staff about ethical issues

    Developing policies and procedures related to ethical issues

    Consulting with staff on ethical issues

    Evaluating the agency's efforts to promote an ethical practice

- Respect and ensure that others respect clients' rights to make informed decisions that conflict with what the health care team believes to be clinically best.

RECOMMENDED READINGS

Adelman RD, Breckman R: Mistreatment. In Abrams WB, Berkow R, editors: *The Merck manual of geriatrics,* Rahway, NJ, 1990, Merck Sharp and Dohme Research Laboratories.

Bahr RT: Selected ethical and legal issues in aging. In Baines EM, editor: *Perspectives on gerontological nursing,* Newbury Park, CA, 1991, SAGE.

Bandman EL, Bandman B: *Nursing ethics through the lifespan,* ed 2, Norwalk, CT, 1990, Appleton and Lange.

Bernzweig EP: *Nurses' liability for malpractice,* ed 5, St Louis, 1990, Mosby.

Calfee BE: Are you restraining your patients right? *Nurs 88* 88(5):148, 1988.

Callahan D: *Setting limits: medical goals in an aging society,* New York, 1987, Simon and Schuster.

Callahan D: *What kind of life: the limits of medical progress,* New York, 1990, Simon and Schuster.

Cournoyer CP: *The nurse manager and the law,* Rockville, MD, 1989, Aspen.

Eliopoulos C: *Legal risks in the long-term care facility,* Glen Arm, MD, 1991, Health Education Network.

Jecker NS, editor: *Aging and ethics,* Clifton, NJ, 1991, Humana Press.

Kane RA, Caplan AL, editors: *Everyday ethics: resolving dilemmas in the nursing home,* New York, 1990, Springer-Verlag.

McConnell LT, Lynn J, Moreno JD: Ethical issues. In Abrams WB, Berkow R, editors: *The Merck manual of geriatrics,* Rahway, NJ, 1990, Merck Sharp and Dohme Research Laboratories.

Regan JL: *Your legal rights in late life,* Glenview, IL, 1989, Scott, Foresman.

Stevenson C, Capezuti E: Guardianship: protection vs. peril, *Geriatr Nurs* 12(1):10, 1991.

Waymack MH, Taler GA: *Medical ethics and the elderly: a case book,* Chicago, 1988, Pluribus.

15

 Services and Resources
for Gerontologic Care

SERVICES

A variety of services are available to promote health and independent function and assist in the management of health and socioeconomic problems of the elderly. Services must be matched to the individual client's needs; two clients with similar health conditions may require significantly different sets of services based on their unique circumstances. Some factors to consider when assessing service needs include the following:

- Physical status
- Mental status
- Health conditions and related care requirements
- Motivation of the client
- Functional capacity for activities of daily living (ADL) and independent activities of daily living (IADL)
- Family resources
- Financial resources
- Living situation, home
- Pattern of self-care
- Preferences regarding care and services
- History of service utilization

Once service needs are identified and services arranged, an ongoing assessment of the appropriateness of services is essential. Changing status of the client or care givers, new self-care demands, loss of financial resources, and other factors can change service needs. Clients should have the ability to flow along the continuum of services as their needs change.

Every state has an agency on aging with local offices that provide information and referral assistance to older adults. Gerontologic nurses should be familiar with these agencies and refer clients to them as appropriate. Also, gerontologic nurses should become familiar with the formal and informal services available in the community to assist clients with locating appropriate resources. Examples of services that can be of benefit are given below.

General

Information and referral. Local libraries, offices on aging, and health departments can direct the client to an appropriate source of help and serve as excellent resources for locating services in a specific community. State health care associations make referrals and are listed in the white pages of telephone books.

Financial aid. Local offices of the Social Security Administration and Department of Social Services determine eligibility for financial assistance and special benefits.

Banking. Transportation and crime problems can be reduced by having Social Security and other checks managed by direct deposit. Many banks offer the elderly free checking and will assist in balancing checkbooks and managing bills.

Recreation. Diversion and activity promote the health and well-being of the elderly. Local bureaus of recreation, religious groups, and service agencies sponsor senior centers and activities. Often theaters, restaurants, and travel agencies provide special discounts for older adults.

Transportation. Public transit agencies and local chapters of the Red Cross can provide or direct the client to low-cost or handicapped transportation. Hospital social work departments may be able to assist with transportation for clinic visits.

Life care. For an initial fee and monthly payment, persons can enter a life-care community that will provide housing and services specific to the interests and needs of older adults. Health care also is included, usually ranging from wellness management through skilled nursing home care. Persons usually enter a life-care community when healthy, with intentions to spend their remaining years there. This arrangement usually provides for housing and various levels of health care as the client's status changes.

When Minimal Assistance is Needed

Homemaker. Public social service and private agencies can provide assistance with light housekeeping and shopping chores to help the elderly maintain independent living in the community.

Assisted living/personal care. Bathing, dressing, and meal assistance may be required by elderly persons who are unable to function with total independence but whose needs do not require continuous assistance or institutionalization. This form of care can be provided within the homes of older adults or their care givers or in designated senior citizen living facilities.

Home-delivered meals. Health departments, social service agencies, and religious organizations can provide or direct the client to such services as Meals on Wheels in a specific community; these will usually provide one warm nutritious meal and a cold snack, delivered right to the client's door.

Foster care. Social service departments can find placement for older persons who need room, board, and supervision in private homes.

Telephone reassurance. Homebound or at-risk elderly can obtain a daily social contact and safety check by having someone call them at a prearranged time.

When Moderate Assistance is Needed

Home health care. A variety of public and private home health agencies may provide this level of service for clients who need skilled nursing services or special therapy, such as physical therapy or dialysis.

Day care/treatment centers. Clients are transported to these sites and receive health, social, and recreational services for a portion of the day. The thrust of the program may be medical, social, or psychiatric.

Hospice. Hospice is an organized approach to the care of terminally ill persons. The goal of this form of care is to provide comfort, caring, and the highest quality of life possible to dying persons and their families. Hospice care offers moderate or total assistance in both community and institutional settings.

When Total Assistance is Needed

Institutional care. Nursing homes, chronic hospitals, and other long-term care facilities offer continuous services to clients when 24-hour care and supervision are needed. These institutions can serve as a permanent or a temporary care site until the client's condition improves.

Combinations. Frequently, very ill individuals can be cared for by the creative combination of multiple resources, such as a day-care program on week-days, homemaker services on week-end days, and a private aide sleeping in during the night. Individual resources and the availability of community resources can determine what the possibilities for these arrangements can be.

The nurse needs to be aware of available resources and plan services carefully, coordinating measures to meet physical, emotional, and socioeconomic needs. Individualized plans are necessary to meet client needs and preferences. Providing preventive, supportive services helps promote independence and can prevent development of problems.

FINANCES

Social Security was developed in 1935 as supplemental income for retired workers in old age. In 1939 the plan changed to include payments to certain dependents when the worker retired and to survivors if the worker died. More participants were allowed in the 1950s such as the self-employed, local and state employees, armed forces, clergy, and household and farm employees. Disability insurance was added in 1954. Cost-of-living provision was enacted in 1972.

- Social Security benefits (based on credits earned during work years)
  - One quarter of coverage is earned for each quarter of worker contribution
  - Special provisions exist for surviving mothers and dependent children of deceased workers who have not earned sufficient credit
  - Dependents of retired, disabled, or deceased workers, unmarried children under 18 years (or 22 years if full-time students); disabled children, dependent spouse over 62 years (or spouse under 62 years caring for dependent children), divorced spouse (under certain conditions)
- Benefit calculation
  - Family benefits based on individual contributions; if both husband and wife qualify, benefits are calculated on the larger of the two amounts
  - A minimum benefit exists
  - Benefits are reduced for retired workers under 72 years

who return to work and earn above a specified
amount

Medicare, a 1965 amendment to the Social Security Act
(Title XVIII), provides medical insurance for persons 65 years or
older. It is a federally funded, standard coverage for all older persons regardless of their state of residence. Payment into the Social
Security system ensures institutional coverage at no cost; physician/outpatient coverage requires payment of a monthly premium. Medicare covers both institutional and physician/outpatient services such as the following:

- Hospital care
- Skilled nursing home care committee
- Hospice care
- Physician services
- Outpatient hospital services
- Outpatient therapies
- Outpatient surgery
- Outpatient rehabilitation

NOTE: Since specific preconditions and limitations may exist for
each service, clients should be advised to consult with an agency's
Medicare resource/specialist or the local office of the Social Security Administration.

Medical Assistance (Medicaid), a 1965 amendment to the
Social Security Act (Title XIX), provides medical insurance to
low-income persons of any age and is funded by state and federal
contributions. For clients eligible for both services, Medical
Assistance supplements Medicare coverage. The services vary
from state to state, but basic coverage includes the following:

- Inpatient hospital care
- Outpatient hospital services
- Laboratory and x-ray services
- Physicians' services
- Nursing home care
- Home health care

Nursing Implications
- Refer clients to the local department of social services to
  determine eligibility and benefits.
- To determine eligibility for various benefits, have clients
  contact the nearest Social Security office when they:
    Are at least 62 years old and within several months of
    retirement

Are 65 years old (retiring or not)
Become disabled
Experience the death of a family member who has
received benefits

ORGANIZATIONS

Many organizations provide educational materials and other
resources pertaining to a specific condition or health problem.
The gerontologic nurse should contact these organizations for
further assistance as needed.

Alcoholism
Al-Anon Family Group Headquarters
1372 Broadway
New York, NY 10018
(212) 302-7240

Alcoholics Anonymous
15 East 26th Street
Room 1817
New York, NY 10010
(212) 683-3900

National Clearinghouse for Alcohol and Drug Information
11426-28 Rockville Pike
Suite 200
Rockville, MD 20852
(800) 729-6686

Alzheimer's Disease
Association for Alzheimer's Disease and Related Disorders
919 North Michigan Avenue
Suite 1000
Chicago, IL 60611
(800) 272-3900

Respite Programs for Caregivers
of Alzheimer's Disease Patients
(Hotline)
(800) 648-COPE

Arthritis
Arthritis Foundation
2045 Peachtree Road NE
Atlanta, GA 30326
(404) 351-0454

Cancer
American Cancer Society
777 Third Avenue
New York, NY 10017
(212) 371-2900

Leukemia Society of America
600 Third Avenue
New York, NY 10016
(212) 473-8484

Make Today Count
PO Box 303
Burlington, IA 52601
(319) 753-6251

National Cancer Institute
Office of Cancer Communications
Building 31, Room 10A18
Bethesda, MD 20205
(800) 492-6600

United Ostomy Association
36 Executive Park
Suite 120
Irvine, CA 92714
(800) 826-0826

Cardiovascular Conditions
American Heart Association
7320 Greenville Avenue
Dallas, TX 75231
(214) 373-6300

High Blood Pressure Information Center
120/80 National Institutes of Health
Bethesda, MD 20205
(301) 496-1809

International Association of Pacemaker Patients
PO Box 54305
Atlanta, GA 30308
(800) 241-6993

Mended Hearts
7320 Greenville Avenue
Dallas, TX 75231

National Amputation Foundation
12-45 150th Street
Whitestone, NY 11357
(212) 767-0596

National Heart, Lung, and Blood Institute
Office of Information
Bethesda, MD 20205

National Stroke Association
8480 East Orchard Road
Suite 1000
Englewood, CO 80111
(800) STROKES

Diabetes
American Diabetes Association
149 Madison Avenue
New York, NY 10016
(212) 725-4925

Diabetes Education Center
4959 Excelsior Boulevard
Minneapolis, MN 55416
(612) 927-3393

National Diabetes Information Clearinghouse
National Institutes of Health
9000 Rockville Pike
Box NDIC
Bethesda, MD 20892
(301) 468-2162

Death and Dying
Choice in Dying
200 Varick Street
10th Floor
New York, NY 10014
(212) 366-5540

Gastrointestinal Conditions
National Foundation for Illeitis and Colitis
295 Madison Avenue
New York, NY 10017
(212) 685-3440

United Ostomy Association
2001 West Beverly Boulevard
Los Angeles, CA 90057
(213) 413-5510

Hearing Impairment
Alexander Graham Bell Association for the Deaf
3417 Volta Place NW
Washington, DC 20007
(202) 337-5220

American Humane Association Hearing Dog Program
1500 West Tufts Avenue
Englewood, CO 80110
(303) 762-0342

National Association for the Deaf
814 Thayer Avenue
Silver Spring, MD 20910
(301) 587-1788

National Center for Law and the Deaf
7th Street and Florida Avenue NE
Washington, DC 20002
(202) 651-5454

Self-Help for Hard of Hearing People
PO Box 34889
Washington, DC 20034

Hospice
National Hospice Organization
North Monroe Street
Suite 901
Arlington, VA 22209
(703) 243-5900

Incontinence
Help for Incontinent People
Box 544
Union, SC 29389
(803) 585-8789

Kimberly Clark Corporation
2001 Marathon Avenue
Neenah, WI 54946
(414) 721-2000

Procter and Gamble
Procter and Gamble Plaza
Cincinnati, OH 45202
(800) 428-8363

Mental Health and Illness
Alcoholics Anonymous
PO Box 459
Grand Central Station
New York, NY 10017
(212) 686-1100

Mental Health Association
1800 North Kent Street
Arlington, VA 22209
(703) 528-6405

Multiple Sclerosis
National Multiple Sclerosis Society
733 Third Avenue
New York, NY 10017
(800) 227-3166

Musculoskeletal Conditions
Arthritis Foundation
3400 Peachtree Road
Suite 1101
Atlanta, GA 30326
(404) 266-0795

Arthritis Information Clearinghouse
PO Box 34427
Bethesda, MD 20034
(301) 881-9411

National Osteoporosis Foundation
1150 17th Street NW
Suite 500
Washington, DC 20036
(202) 223-2226

Nursing Homes
Nursing Home Information Service Center
National Council of Senior Citizens
1331 F Street
Suite 500
Washington, DC 20004
(202) 347-8800

Pain
American Pain Society
5700 Old Orchard Road
Skokie, IL 60077
(708) 966-5595

National Chronic Pain Outreach Association
8222 Wycliff Court
Manassas, VA 22110
(703) 368-7357

Parkinson's Disease
American Parkinson's Disease Association
116 John Street
New York, NY 10038
(212) 732-9550

National Parkinson Foundation
1501 NW 9th Avenue
Miami, FL 33136
(305) 547-6666

Parkinson's Disease Foundation
William Black Medical Research Building
640-650 West 168th Street
New York, NY 10032
(212) 923-4700

Parkinson Support Group of American
11376 Cherry Hill Road
Suite 204
Beltsville, MD 20705
(301) 937-1545

United Parkinson Foundation
360 W. Superior Street
Chicago, IL 60610
(312) 664-2344

Pulmonary Conditions
American Lung Association
1740 Broadway
New York, NY 10019
(212) 315-8700

Asthma and Allergy Foundation of America
1125 15th Street NW
Suite 502
Washington, DC 20005
(202) 466-7643

Emphysema Anonymous
PO Box 66
Fort Myers, FL 33902
(813) 334-4226

Visual Impairment
American Council of the Blind
1156 15th Street NW
Suite 720
Washington, DC 20005
(800) 424-8666

Blinded Veterans Association
1735 DeSales Street NW
Washington, DC 20036
(202) 347-4010

Guide Dogs for the Blind
PO Box 1200
San Rafael, CA 94902
(415) 479-4000

Guiding Eyes for the Blind
611 Granite Springs Road
Yorktown Heights, NY 10598
(800) 942-0149

Leader Dogs for the Blind
1039 South Rochester Road
Rochester, MN 48063
(313) 651-9011

National Association for the Visually Handicapped
3201 Balboa Street
San Francisco, CA 94121
(415) 221-3201

National Eye Institute
Building 31, Room 6A-32
Bethesda, MD 20205
(301) 496-5248

National Federation of the Blind
1800 Johnson Street
Baltimore, MD 21230
(410) 659-9314

National Library Service for the Blind and Physically Handicapped
Library of Congress
1291 Taylor Street NW
Washington, DC 20542
(202) 287-5100

Recorded Periodicals
919 Walnut Street
Philadelphia, PA 19107
(215) 627-0600

Recordings for the Blind
215 West 58th Street
New York, NY 10022
(212) 751-0860

Index

Numerals in italic refer to illustrations. Numerals followed by a "t" refer to tables.